Seizures AND Epilepsy IN Children

A JOHNS HOPKINS PRESS HEALTH BOOK

Seizures AND Epilepsy IN Children

A COMPREHENSIVE GUIDE

4TH EDITION

Eileen P. G. Vining, MD ◆ Sarah C. Doerrer, MS, CPNP

Christa W. Habela, MD, PhD ◆ Adam L. Hartman, MD

Sarah A. Kelley, MD ◆ Eric H. Kossoff, MD ◆ Cynthia F. Salorio, PhD

Samata Singhi, MD, MSc ◆ Carl E. Stafstrom, MD, PhD

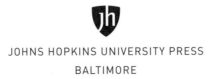

JOHNS HOPKINS UNIVERSITY PRESS

BALTIMORE

Note to the Reader: This book is not meant to substitute for medical care, and treatment should not be based solely on its contents. Instead, treatment must be developed in a dialogue between the individual and their physician. Our book has been written to help with that dialogue.

Drug dosage: The author and publisher have made reasonable efforts to determine that the selection of drugs discussed in this text conform to the practices of the general medical community. The medications described do not necessarily have specific approval by the US Food and Drug Administration for use in the diseases for which they are recommended. In view of ongoing research, changes in governmental regulation, and the constant flow of information relating to drug therapy and drug reactions, the reader is urged to check the package insert of each drug for any change in indications and dosage and for warnings and precautions. This is particularly important when the recommended agent is a new and/or infrequently used drug.

Johns Hopkins University Press
2715 North Charles Street
Baltimore, Maryland 21218
www.press.jhu.edu

Figure 1.1 is used courtesy of iStock photo. Figures 1.2–1.5, 2.1–2.7, and 10.1 are by Timothy H. Phelps. Figures 1.6 and 14.1 are by Jane Whitney. Figure 7.1 is used courtesy of Nihon Kohden. Figure 7.10 is by Keith Weller, © The Johns Hopkins Hospital.

Special discounts are available for bulk purchases of this book.
For more information, please contact Special Sales at specialsales@jh.edu.

The last printed page of the book is a continuation of this copyright page.

Contents

Part III. Treatment

Seizures AND Epilepsy IN Children

Introduction

Many families whose children have had a single seizure, and many others whose children have epilepsy, come to us for a second opinion. There are common themes among all these families. One theme is that the family and child are focused on the seizure or seizures; they are unable to look at the whole child and the bigger picture. Their life and their child's life have become centered primarily on the seizures. A second theme is that the families and children are overwhelmed by the mythology of epilepsy, by the fear of future disability or intellectual disability. Few families understand what seizures are and what they are not. They come seeking to understand what has happened and what is likely to happen.

Many physicians, even those very knowledgeable about seizures, epilepsy, and their treatment, focus on these medical aspects and do not put epilepsy in the proper perspective of the whole child and family. We believe that no child's life should be defined by seizures. No one is "an epileptic." The seizures and epilepsy are often only a small portion of the child's life. We believe that to put them in perspective you must understand the brain, seizures, and how to cope with epilepsy. You must understand the mythology and how different it often is from reality. Only with this understanding can you avoid unnecessarily disabling your child, prevent them being limited by others, and allow them to reach their full potential. That is why we have written this book and why we continue to revise it. While primarily for parents, it is also a book for everyone with seizures and for all who are touched by seizures—families, teachers, and health professionals.

We hope this book will reassure you that a majority of children who have epilepsy can have their seizures completely controlled with medication and can function well in school and in their future lives. Many of these children will, after a time, stop taking medicine and will have outgrown their epilepsy. For some parents whose children's epilepsy has not been completely controlled or whose children have atypical development or disabling conditions, we hope our book will help you and them to function as normally as possible and to maximize their assets and minimize their disabilities.

Parents come to us with many fears: "Will my child be all right?" "Will he swallow his tongue?" "Will she die?" "Does she have a brain tumor?" "Will he be intellectually disabled?" "Can he ever lead a normal life?" "Can seizures ever be controlled?" "Can I ever leave her alone?" "Will medication make him an addict?" All these thoughts, and more, run through the mind of a parent whose child has had a seizure. The children themselves have similar fears: "Is this going to happen again?" "What will my friends think?" "Will I ever be able to ride my bike again?" "Can I go to college?" "Can I ever drive?" "Will I be able to get married?" "What about having children?"

Before we can help you to deal with these fears and put epilepsy in perspective, we must debunk the mythology. Both terms, epilepsy and seizures, carry the myths and misconceptions of centuries past, when people who experienced them were thought to be possessed by witches or devils and were confined in special colonies or shunned. People saw a child suddenly "seized," losing control, falling to the floor, his body jerking. A few minutes later this child was back to normal. What could have caused this to happen? It must have been some outside force! The devil? Not so long ago people believed this. We now know that seizures come from electrical disruptions in the brain.

Also part of the mythology, many people still believe that epilepsy and seizures are always devastating, that they will continue to recur, that they will get worse, that the brain will be damaged, and that their child might become disabled, intellectually limited, or even die. Now we know that only some children who have a single seizure have a second seizure. We also now know that most children who have had several seizures, who by definition have epilepsy, will still have their seizures controlled with medication, and that most children outgrow their seizures and can be taken off medication. Only a minority of children with epilepsy will have difficult-to-control seizures. Most children with seizures are quite normal all or virtually all the time, except during the seizure.

The folk tales persist because epilepsy remains a hidden condition. People see only the small percentage of children who are severely disabled and have seizures. The vast majority, whose seizures are well controlled and who function well, do not advertise that they have epilepsy. If your neighbor's child has seizures and is doing well, you may never even know that the child has epilepsy. Only if they have a seizure when their friends are around do the friends become aware of the child's epilepsy. Their friends' parents may say, "I never knew they had epilepsy. They look so normal!" "I thought that all children with epilepsy were disabled." "The only child I knew with seizures was in a wheelchair and never went to school." If we want to combat these old myths and prejudices, children with epilepsy and their families have to be far more comfortable and open about the disorder. Only then will the public understand that most people with epilepsy are just like themselves. Seeing only children with epilepsy who are disabled, you get the wrong impression. You may have no idea that most children who have epilepsy live almost normal and very productive and fulfilling lives. You can limit your child if you continue to believe the myths.

Most individuals with epilepsy can function normally, becoming exuberant children, vigorous adolescents, and productive adults who are free of seizures altogether. Yet we still see children limited when they are young by parental overprotection. You will have to learn what protections are reasonable and realistic, and which restrictions will simply handicap your child. Avoiding overprotection will require that you understand not only seizures but also your reaction to them, your child's reaction, and the reactions of others. You need to work actively to prevent seizures from becoming a handicap. In most cases, you can succeed. Society's misperceptions and prejudices can handicap your child. The Epilepsy Foundation (EF), the national voluntary organization for people with epilepsy, has done a wonderful job over the past decades of informing the public of the truth about epilepsy and about people with epilepsy. EF has attempted to dispel the prejudice embodied in the term "epileptic" and has advocated strongly that we eliminate this word from our vocabulary. But prejudice can't be wholly eliminated with words and information alone. Prejudice must be fought by example as well. To overcome your prejudice truly, you have to play with children who have epilepsy; you have to go to school with them, live with them, and come to realize that they are children just like other children, with their own strengths and weaknesses, peculiarities, and personality. They just happen to have seizures.

Not every child or adult with epilepsy will avoid disabilities. Some are handicapped by brain damage from head trauma, infection, or the other multiple causes of epilepsy. Others are affected by intellectual or motor impairment. Some are disabled by their difficult-to-control seizures, despite many new medications. For all persons with epilepsy, better understanding and services continue to be needed and will improve their lives. In many areas local EF affiliates can provide information, resources, and programs. They can be an important source of support for families of children with epilepsy.

If children believe in the mythology, they can limit themselves. If they allow themselves to be overprotected, if they believe they can't do things because of their seizures, then they will be unable to reach their full potential. Just as you must allow them to take risks, so they must be willing to try new things. It requires self-esteem, courage, and determination for them to venture into the unknown, to stay at another child's house when it's possible they could have another seizure, to go to the school dance when they might be embarrassed, to apply for a job when a seizure could occur and someone might find out that they have epilepsy. Once disabled by fear of seizures or by overprotection, a child has difficulty breaking free and leading a normal life. It is far easier to prevent a disability than to overcome it.

Helping your child to reach their full potential will require a partnership between you and your child's physician. This book will help you create that. For example, your child's physician will do tests and may propose medication, but do not allow the physician to make all the decisions. Your doctor should be familiar with epilepsy, with the choice of medications for controlling seizures, and with their side effects. They should be willing to discuss with you the risks and benefits of each medication and of each test, but it is your job, as the parent, to be a partner in the management—to be an informed consumer. You should ask: "Why is this test being done?" "What are its risks?" "What are the risks and benefits of treatment?" As a parent, you will be your child's best advocate if you are informed and understand seizures and their treatment. You must understand what epilepsy is and what it is not. You must understand what is fiction and what is fact.

We have written this book to help you understand seizures, your reaction to them, and the reaction of others. Through the stories of many of our patients, we illustrate how accurate diagnosis, comprehensive treatment and management, and sensitivity to the impact of seizures can help a child and their family live better with epilepsy. With medical information, you will understand the many different kinds of seizures, how the brain is organized, and how it works. With knowledge of medications and other therapies, you will understand your child's treatment. With actual knowledge of the learning and behavioral problems that can occur, you will optimize their comprehensive management. Only with this more complete understanding can you become a strong advocate on the team that is helping your child.

PART I

Why Do Seizures AND Epilepsy Occur?

CHAPTER 1

How the Brain Works
Keys to Understanding Seizures and Epilepsy

As the parent or caretaker of a child with recently diagnosed seizures or epilepsy, you may be anxious about your child's diagnosis and have questions such as what a seizure is, how a seizure differs from epilepsy, and possible complications of seizures and their treatment. We believe that parents and children should be participants in their own care. To be an effective participant, it helps to be knowledgeable about how the brain works. Our goal is to demystify seizures and epilepsy and provide you with useful information to educate yourself, be able to explain what's going on to your child, discuss your child's diagnosis with relatives and friends, and ask appropriate questions when visiting your child's doctors and other professionals. Armed with this knowledge, you will hopefully come to see seizures as less scary and more manageable. This introductory chapter first discusses how the normal brain functions and then explains that a seizure represents a temporary disruption of normal brain activity. By understanding some basic information about the anatomy of the brain (its structure) and its physiology (how it works) you will better appreciate many of the different types of seizures that occur, why they happen, and why certain treatments are recommended.

Normal Brain Structure

The brain is composed of several parts, each having a different function (Figure 1.1). Large sections of the brain are known as lobes. The frontal lobe controls movement, thinking, imagination, and decision making, while other lobes enable us to talk and interpret what we see, hear, and feel. Each lobe of the brain comprises millions and millions of cells called neurons that work together as a network. Each neuron communicates with many neighboring neurons as well as with cells in distant areas of the brain. The neuron network is somewhat like a society. Like a human society, brain neurons usually cooperate and function quite normally. When neurons do not function normally, the result might be a seizure.

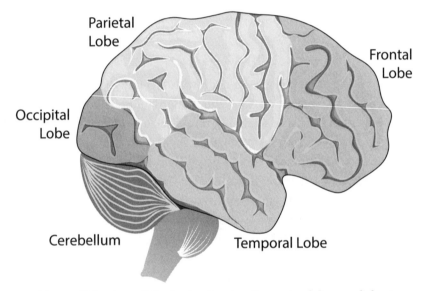

FIGURE 1.1. Side view of the brain showing the major lobes, each having a different function. The frontal lobe controls movement and thinking, such as making decisions. The parietal lobe processes sensation. Temporal lobe functions include memory processing and emotion. The occipital lobe is responsible for interpreting visual images. The cerebellum modulates coordination.

Normal Brain Function

Neurons communicate with each other by *firing*, which means that they use tiny amounts of electrical activity to transmit information from one cell to another. This biological electrical activity is minute compared to the electricity that, say, runs our computers or home appliances. Yet, the tiny electrical impulses generated at the cell body of a neuron (Figure 1.2) travel to other neurons, both near and far, providing the instructions for us to move, think, and experience or display emotions.

Neurons transmit their electrical impulses along conducting "wires" called *axons* (Figure 1.2). An electrical impulse generated in the cell body of a neuron travels down its axon to the synapse, which is a narrow gap between neurons. The electrical impulse causes the release of a chemical called a neurotransmitter from the synaptic terminal of one neuron onto the next neuron, where the neurotransmitter either "excites" the next neuron (makes it fire impulses) or "inhibits" it (prevents it from firing) (Figure 1.3). That is, some neurotransmitters excite and others inhibit the firing of other neurons. The brain needs both excitatory activity and inhibitory activity to function properly.

Neurons that cause excitation and neurons that cause inhibition

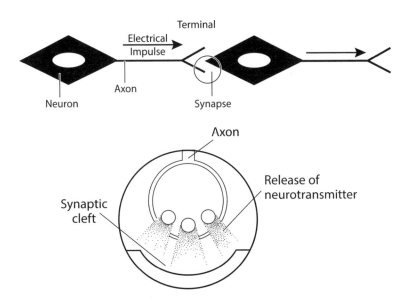

FIGURE 1.2. Communication between neurons. Neurons communicate by tiny electrical impulses that travel from the cell body along the axon to the synaptic terminal, from which a chemical called a neurotransmitter is released in response to the electrical impulse. The neurotransmitter flows across a small gap between neurons called a synapse, onto the next neuron. A neurotransmitter either excites or inhibits the next neuron.

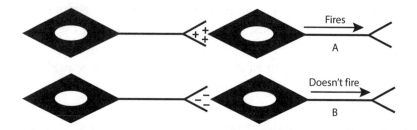

FIGURE 1.3. Neuronal excitation and inhibition in the brain. Some neurotransmitters, released by a neuron, excite a neighboring neuron (+), causing it to fire (*A*). Other neurotransmitters inhibit the next cell (−) and make it less likely to fire (*B*). The balance between excitatory (+) and inhibitory (−) impulses that reach each neuron determines whether it will fire onto the next neuron in a network. Excessive excitation could lead to seizure activity. The goal of anti-seizure medicines and other treatments is to restore the excitation/inhibition balance in the brain.

are intermixed and interconnected in all parts of the brain. To move a finger, for example, a certain number of neurons must be activated, or excited, in the area of the brain's frontal lobe devoted to finger control; this excitation instructs finger muscle fibers to contract. If a group of cells in that area fire excessively, however, with too much excitation, uncontrolled twitching of the hand may occur. That sometimes happens in a seizure.

If, for some reason, there is too much excitatory activity or too little inhibitory activity in one part of the brain or in the whole brain, then the balance of excitation and inhibition is disrupted, and a seizure could occur (Figure 1.4). The amount of excitation needed for a seizure to occur is called the *seizure threshold*.

Typically, the brain is stable, and the balance between excitation and inhibition is carefully regulated. The mechanisms controlling the stability of brain activity have been compared to driving a car with one foot on the accelerator ("excites" the car's movement) and the other foot on the brake (inhibits the car's movement). The vehicle's speed and function will depend on how much pressure is exerted on the accelerator and how much pressure is exerted on the brake. It's the balance that counts!

Threshold

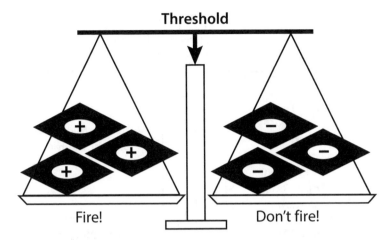

Fire!   Don't fire!

FIGURE 1.4. Neuron firing threshold is the balance between excitatory (+) and inhibitory (−) influences. A loss of inhibition or an increase in excitatory influences (or both!) may cause a neuron to reach its threshold and fire. Similarly, a loss of excitation or an increase in inhibition may cause a cell not to fire.

What Triggers a Seizure? The Concept of Seizure Threshold

Many cells must be firing at the same time for a seizure to occur. As discussed above, the excitation and inhibition in the brain are normally in balance. If excitation gets large enough (or inhibition gets small enough), due to various genetic, medical, or environmental factors, seizure "threshold" is reached, and a seizure occurs. Things like stress, fever, illness, or insufficient sleep can all lower the threshold for a seizure in a person prone to seizures. These stressors can "tip the balance" of brain activity toward too much excitation (hyperexcitable), leading to the seizure, which can be envisioned as the electrical messages between neurons becoming jumbled. Our attempts to prevent or treat seizures, using medications or other measures, aim to decrease the excitation or increase the inhibition of neuron firing. That is, we try to raise the threshold for abnormal firing of neurons (increase the "margin of safety"). The threshold for a seizure depends on many factors, especially genetics (Figure 1.5). Consider this case example.

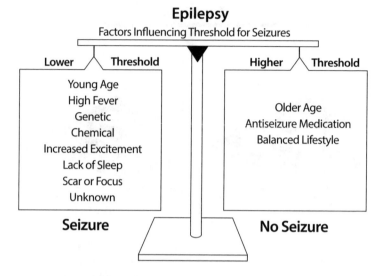

FIGURE 1.5. Seizure threshold is the amount of summated excitation that leads to excessive neuron firing and generation of a seizure in the neuron network. Factors influencing seizure threshold are illustrated here.

Ms. Jones was driving her son Lamar and his friend Michael to school when a truck rear ended her car. Both children were seat-belted in the backseat, but the impact caused them to lurch forward and hit their heads against the front seats. Michael had a tonic-clonic seizure. Lamar did not have a seizure and was fine except for a bump on his head.

Why did one boy have a seizure and the other not? One possibility was that Michael hit his head harder and this caused a greater disturbance of brain activity. A second possibility is that Michael may be genetically prone to seizures and may have a lower seizure threshold. Therefore, although each boy had a head injury of similar severity, in Michael's case, the head trauma was sufficient to trigger a seizure.

Young children have lower seizure thresholds than adults. That is why young children may have a seizure when they get a fever (febrile seizure, see Chapter 4), but adults do not. Febrile seizures tend to run in families and disappear when the child is 4 or 5 years old. Emotional and other physical factors also affect seizure threshold. Excitement in response to a birthday party or trip; agitation caused by an argument, excitement, or punishment; or anxiety during an exam can all lower an individual's threshold, or *margin of safety*, and lead to a seizure. Lack of sufficient sleep is a major trigger for seizures. Chemical changes in the blood, such as low blood sugar or low calcium levels, may likewise make neurons more susceptible to firing and lead to a seizure. Anyone can have a seizure if a trauma or other brain disturbance exceeds their threshold at a given time. Antiseizure medicines are designed to increase the margin of safety and decrease the chance of a seizure occurring. If someone forgets to take their seizure medicine, the margin of safety decreases, and a seizure becomes more likely.

What Is a Seizure?

So what exactly is a seizure, and is it the same as epilepsy? To begin our discussion, see the definition of several important terms in Table 1.1. There are many types of seizures, ranging from a staring spell lasting a few seconds (during which a child may not respond to their name being called), to a convulsion involving stiffening and shaking of one or both arms or legs. Types of seizures are discussed in depth in Chapter 2. Here, it is important to understand that a seizure is a single event, caused by sudden, abnormal electrical discharges in the brain that result in an alteration in behavior, movement, sensation, or consciousness. Any of us could have a seizure in a certain situation, such as immediately following a head injury, in the course of a brain infection such as meningitis, or as an adverse response to certain medicines, toxins, or drugs. A single seizure does not mean epilepsy, and many people have only one seizure in their lifetime. Epilepsy is diagnosed when seizures occur repeatedly over time.

Epilepsy Is More than Seizures

Some people use the term *seizure disorder* as a substitute for epilepsy. This term should not be used. Epilepsy does involve seizures, of course, but much more. If epilepsy is thought about as an iceberg (Figure 1.6), seizures would be like the tip of the iceberg—they are visible to observers just as the iceberg is visible above the water's surface. A child with epilepsy must deal with having seizures, often at unpredictable times.

TABLE 1.1. Important Definitions

Seizure A single episode of abnormal brain firing, causing a person to experience altered neurologic function. This may involve abnormal awareness, changes in the ability to talk or understand speech, rhythmic motor movements, abnormal sensations, or changes in vital signs such as heart rate or breathing rate.

Epilepsy The term epilepsy is used when a person has experienced two or more unprovoked seizures more than 24 hours apart, or a single seizure with more than a 60% chance or recurrence, or the diagnosis of an epilepsy syndrome. In epilepsy, seizures can occur unexpectedly, often without warning.

Seizure disorder This term should not be used. The term epilepsy is more meaningful and helps us think about all the other issues that must be addressed in caring for the child.

Epilepsy syndrome When features of a child's epilepsy match those of other children with similar seizure type(s), age of onset, EEG findings, responsiveness to certain medicines or other treatments, and other aspects, as discussed in the text (Chapter 8), an epilepsy syndrome is diagnosed.

Seizure focus An area of the brain that generates seizure activity. The focus might be a small scar or area of the brain that did not form properly during prenatal development, or sometimes no abnormality of brain structure can be identified, on imaging or EEG studies, to explain the focus.

Yet, persons with epilepsy may also need to deal with other challenges that might affect daily life but are not as obvious (these challenges are like the part of the iceberg below the water's surface).

These challenges include the need to take medications regularly and possible side effects of those medicines, the psychological and social complications around having seizures, and how being prone to having seizures might affect activities such as playing sports, going to sleepovers, and riding a bicycle. Some, but by no means all, children with epilepsy have a higher risk of anxiety, depression, learning difficul-

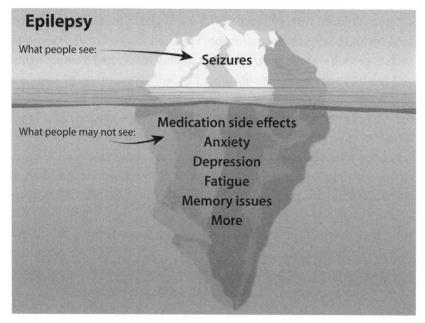

FIGURE 1.6. Seizures can be envisioned as "the tip of the iceberg" in epilepsy. Other medical and psychosocial aspects of epilepsy (below the surface) might pose challenges for persons with epilepsy.

ties, and other so-called comorbidities. All these topics, and how best to deal with them, are discussed later in this book.

Explaining to Your Child How the Brain Works and Why a Seizure Happens

A child's understanding of how the brain works will depend on their age and cognitive level. Likewise, the explanation of why they have a seizure will be based on their level of understanding. Most children understand that light bulbs operate by electricity. Similarly, the brain works by tiny electrical signals. When a light bulb flickers, proper electricity is not flowing through the electrical circuit. Similarly, when a seizure occurs, the brain's electrical signals are temporarily jumbled and not working properly. Most of the time, our electronic devices and our brains work just fine, and children with epilepsy should not be considered "abnormal."

True, children with epilepsy may need to take a medicine to prevent seizures and be especially careful about possible triggers of their seizures, such as getting enough sleep, avoiding alcohol intake and flashing lights, and taking their medicines on time. But with appropriate precautions and proper treatment, most children with epilepsy can participate in the majority of childhood activities with their peers. Prognosis, or long-term outcome, of seizures depends on what kind of epilepsy a child has. It is often difficult to predict, especially at first, when a child's seizures will occur and when and if they will go away. Parents need to be honest with their child. If a parent doesn't know an answer to their child's question or doesn't know how to explain something, they should tell their child that they will find the information for them. Parents should try to address their child's concerns and fears with appropriate optimism and reassurance. Over time, some of these uncertainties become clearer. These topics are discussed more fully in subsequent chapters.

CHAPTER 2

The Kinds of Seizures and Where They Arise in the Brain

Episodic electrical events can occur in different areas of the brain, and the type of seizure they produce will differ depending on what area is affected. Basically, anything the brain can do as a function, it also can do as a seizure.

The Many Types of Seizures

• *You heard a loud noise and ran to Malik's room. Your son was stiff, his back was arched, he didn't seem to be breathing, and he was turning blue. Then he started shaking violently and was foaming at the mouth. Your first thought was that he was about to die!*

• *Maria was sitting with you at the dinner table when suddenly she stopped eating and stared into space. You called her, but she didn't respond. You had to call her several times. "Why does she daydream so often?" you wondered.*

• *Billy comes running to you with a frightened look on his face. He is pale and then has a glassy look in his eyes. You call him, but he doesn't respond. You notice that he is smacking his lips and fumbling with his clothes. Then as you hold him, he stiffens and begins to shake violently.*

• *Michiko began to have jerking at the corner of her mouth. "It's just a habit," her doctor had said, but it's gotten worse. Now the jerking is there all the time, and sometimes it spreads to involve the whole side of her face.*

All the events described above are seizures, and yet each differs from the others. Each may require a different evaluation by your child's physician. Each may require different medication. Each may have a different outcome. The type of seizure depends largely on where in the brain it starts and on the direction and speed of the spread of electrical activity.

Seizures are divided into two major groups, *focal* seizures and *generalized* seizures. Focal seizures begin in one part of the brain. Identifying focal seizures is important, because they may indicate a problem in a specific area of the brain, which might need special attention. The physician looks for an abnormality, such as an area that did not develop normally, a scar, a tangle of blood vessels, or a tumor as the cause of this type of seizure. If focal seizures are not controlled with medication, then surgery can be considered. Generalized seizures, on the other hand, seem to start over diffuse areas of the brain on both sides all at once.

Because the diagnosis of a seizure is based on a history of the event—the history you and other witnesses give—your description is critical to the physician's assessment. Witnessing a seizure is stressful, and you may not be able to recall all the details, such as which way the eyes moved, which limb shook, and how long the shaking lasted. If the episode recurs, then careful observation, particularly at the beginning of the event, or better yet, a video of the event, may be extremely valuable. A movie is worth a thousand words to the physician who is trying to understand what has happened.

When seizures start focally, in a particular area of the brain, and when they spread slowly enough, in seconds or minutes, their onset can be experienced and witnessed or remembered, as in Billy's case.

How do focal seizures spread to other areas of the brain? Why don't all focal seizures spread? What keeps a focal seizure limited to one area? We are only starting to understand this process, and we do not have enough answers to apply to our patients yet. Generalized seizures have no identifiable focal onset, and we are only starting to understand the circuitry of how they start.

Terms Describing the Phases of a Seizure

Physicians commonly use certain special terms to describe parts of a seizure: *aura, ictus,* and *postictal.*

Aura. An aura is simply the start of a small focal seizure. The frightened feeling that Billy experienced is called an aura if it precedes a bigger seizure. If the feeling is all that Billy experiences, he is said to have had an aura—a *focal seizure.* This may be the warning of a more widespread seizure to come. If the seizure spreads within the temporal lobe and affects consciousness, then it becomes a *focal impaired awareness seizure.* If it spreads throughout the brain, resulting in stiffening and generalized shaking, it becomes a *bilateral tonic-clonic seizure.* But with each seizure, the onset, which may be an abnormal smell, taste, abdominal sensation, or emotion (its focal beginning), is still called the aura.

Ictus. Ictus is the Latin word for "stroke" or "attack." Physicians sometimes use the word to mean a seizure.

Postictal. Postictal means "after the attack" or seizure. After a person has had a seizure involving motor activity of the arm, the arm may be weak or even paralyzed for minutes or hours. This is termed a *postictal paralysis,* also called Todd's paralysis, after the physician who identified it. After a generalized tonic-clonic seizure, the person may go to sleep for a period. This is one example of a postictal state. After a focal seizure, the person may have postictal confusion. Each of these conditions occurs *after* the seizure is over.

When observers say, "This person's seizure lasted an hour," what they really mean is that the individual had a generalized tonic-clonic seizure, which may have lasted only two minutes, but that the person then slept (was in a postictal state) for an hour. The difference between the two is important, because there is *little* danger from the postictal state. That quiescent state is simply the time necessary for the brain to recover and return to its normal functioning. If the seizure (jerking) had lasted for the entire hour, that would have been considered a medical emergency.

How Are Seizures Classified?

The Old System: Grand Mal and Petit Mal Seizures
At one time, seizures were classified into two types: big and small—in French, *grand* and *petit*. Since seizures were thought of as bad—*mal* in French—they were classified as *grand mal* and *petit mal*, terms still, unfortunately, used by many patients and physicians. It is unfortunate because they are imprecise. Many types of seizures are "big and bad," causing a patient to fall to the ground and shake. Malik's seizure and Billy's seizure caused each child to fall down and shake, so in the old days, both would have been called *grand mal* seizures. But the two seizures were different; Billy's seizure had a focal beginning.

The term *grand mal* (big and bad) means different things to different people. Some people consider big a seizure that another, with worse seizures, might consider small. If one person has a spell in which she just stops and stares, as Maria did, while another, like Billy, has a spell in which he stares, smacks his lips, and is confused, and a third, such as Michiko, has jerking of the face—are these little spells all petit mal? They are different types of seizures, coming from different parts of the brain, with different implications of causation, requiring different evaluation and different medications, and probably having differing outcomes. Thus, the terms *grand mal* and *petit mal* are now seldom used in classifying seizures.

The New System: Generalized and Focal Seizures
An internationally accepted system of classification of seizures was adopted in 2017 (Table 2.1). This new classification separates seizures into *generalized, focal,* and unknown based on the onset of the seizure.

Focal seizures may or may not alter consciousness or awareness, depending on where they start and which structures of the brain they involve. Focal seizures that do *not* alter consciousness are called *focal aware seizures,* but in the past, they were called *partial, focal motor,* or *focal sensory* seizures. Focal seizures in which consciousness is altered or lost are called *focal impaired awareness seizures.*

Generalized seizures affect diffuse areas of both sides of the brain,

TABLE 2.1. Seizure Classification

International classification	Old term
Focal seizures	Partial or local seizures
Focal onset: aware (consciousness not impaired) *or* impaired awareness (consciousness impaired)	Simple partial or complex partial seizures (psychomotor seizures)
Motor onset	With motor symptoms
Automatisms	
Atonic	Akinetic, drop attacks
Clonic	
Epileptic spasms	
Hyperkinetic	Hypermotor
Myoclonic	
Tonic	
Nonmotor onset	Focal sensory
Autonomic	With autonomic symptoms
Behavior arrest	
Cognitive	
Emotional	With psychic symptoms
Sensory	With somatosensory symptoms
Focal to bilateral tonic-clonic	Partial that secondarily generalize

Generalized onset seizures

Motor
Tonic-clonic
Clonic
Tonic
Myoclonic
Myoclonic-tonic-clonic
Myoclonic-atonic
Atonic
Epileptic spasms *(cont.)*

TABLE 2.1. Seizure Classification, continued

International classification	Old term
Generalized onset seizures (cont.)	
Nonmotor	
Typical	
Atypical	Partial that secondarily generalize
Myoclonic	
Eyelid myoclonia	
Tonic-clonic	
Unknown onset seizures	
Motor	
Tonic-clonic	
Epileptic spasms	
Motor	
Behavior arrest	
Unclassified	

SOURCE: Adapted from *Epilepsia* 58 (2017): 522-30.

not just one part, and they alter consciousness. In a generalized seizure, there is no obvious focal onset or aura. When there is a focal onset, and the seizure progresses to involve the whole brain, it is termed a *focal to bilateral tonic-clonic seizure.*

Generalized seizures can be convulsive or nonconvulsive. *Nonconvulsive* refers to alterations of consciousness without jerking movements. *Convulsive* here means that there are muscle movements like jerking or stiffening.

Focal Seizures and the Anatomy of the Brain

To understand focal seizures and their many manifestations, it is necessary to understand something about the anatomy of the brain. Indeed, it was from a careful study of the events that occurred during focal seizures that Dr. Hughlings Jackson, considered the father of modern understandings of epilepsy, first deduced the organization of the brain. He watched the slow spread of focal seizures (subsequently called Jacksonian seizures) from the finger to the hand to the arm and then to the face, and reasoned that these areas must be next to one another in the brain. The result was the identification of the anatomy of the motor strip (Figure 2.1).

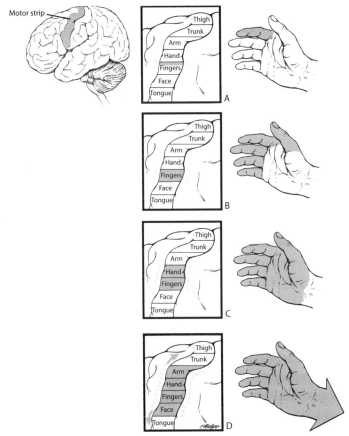

FIGURE 2.1. Brain, showing motor strip and progression of motor symptoms of a focal-onset seizure. Hughlings Jackson observed the slow spread of seizures from the jerking of a finger (*A*), to the jerking of all fingers (*B*), to involvement of the hand and wrist (*C*), then arm and face (*D*). From this spread, he deduced the anatomy of the motor strip of the brain. Hence, seizures of this sort have been called Jacksonian seizures.

These deductions were subsequently confirmed by Dr. Wilder Pen-field and Dr. Herbert Jasper, who, during operations to remove tissue responsible for focal epilepsy, stimulated areas of the brain with small amounts of electricity. Depending on which area was stimulated, a finger would move, a foot would jerk, the face and tongue would twitch, or a finger or lip would tingle. Even certain memories or images would be recalled. Minute electrical stimulation is used today to "map the brain" before a surgeon removes electrically abnormal brain tissue, so that tissue important to normal function can be identified and avoided during the surgery (see Chapter 14).

As the human brain has evolved, its thinking and processing parts have grown in size and complexity. The "thinking" part of the brain is the neocortex. The neocortex (referred to hereafter as the cortex) has four major sections, called lobes, each responsible for separate func-tions (Figure 2.2). The frontal lobes are responsible for personality and memory. The temporal lobes on the left side control speech (in most

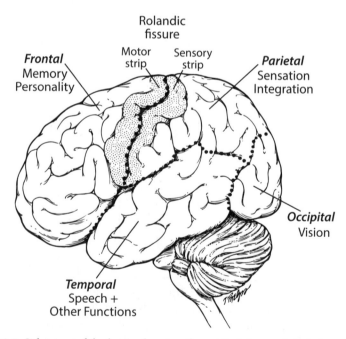

Figure 2.2. Side view of the brain showing the major lobes and their functions, as well as the motor and sensory strips.

TABLE 2.2. Localization of Function within the Brain

Function	Area	Left side	Right side	Deficit if removed
Motor	Motor strip	Control of face, arm, and leg on right side of body	Control of face, arm, and leg on left side of body	Weakness (hemiparesis) of the opposite side
Sensory	Sensory strip	Sensation from right side of body	Sensation from left side of body	Inability to identify what is in hand, where hand is in space, whom hand belongs to, and so on
Cortical sensation	Parietal lobe	Integration of sensation from right side of body	Integration of sensation from left side of body	
Vision	Occipital lobe	Vision to the right side of the body	Vision to the left side of the body	Lack of vision of things to one side or the other
Speech	Temporal lobe	Speech (on left side in 95% of right-handed people; on left side in 70% of left-handed people)		
Intelligence, personality, sense of humor	Not lateralized or localized			

people), and those on the right control subtle higher functions, such as spatial and musical recognition. The parietal lobes contain areas for making associations and interpreting sensations, such as the ability to recognize objects placed in the hand. The occipital lobes are the site of processing visual information.

The *left* side of the brain controls movements of the *right* side of the body and receives sensation from the *right* side of the body. Thus, the left occipital lobe processes vision of things in your right field of vision, and the *right* side of the brain processes similar functions for the left side of the body (Table 2.2).

The temporal lobes and the frontal lobes are the most important in a discussion of epilepsy because they are the most *epileptogenic*. These regions are densely packed with neurons and have very wide connections to other parts of the brain, which may partly account for why so many seizures start in this area of the brain.

Motor and Sensory Areas

Perhaps the easiest areas of the brain to understand and explain are the motor strip and sensory strip (Figure 2.3). If a surgeon were to remove a person's skull and the coverings of the brain to expose the motor strip of the frontal lobe and introduce a small amount of electrical current (stimulus) on the brain surface in the finger area (area 1), the awake patient might see some twitching of the index finger of one hand. If this were done to the left side of the brain, the right index finger might twitch. Were the surgeon to move the current slightly up or down the strip, it might cause another finger to move. Moving the current to the face area (2) would cause facial movements; in area 3, the arm on the right side of the body might jerk. These movements are, in a sense, little seizures, a slight seizure induced by the surgeon's electrical stimulus.

If the electrical stimulus comes from within the brain cells themselves (rather than from a surgeon's electrical stimulus), caused, for example, by an abnormally developed part of the brain, a scar, a stroke, or a tumor, the resulting movement would be called a seizure. If the seizure stays local (focal), it may consist of just the repeated twitch of a finger, a hand, or the face. If the seizure focus is in the sensory strip and occurs

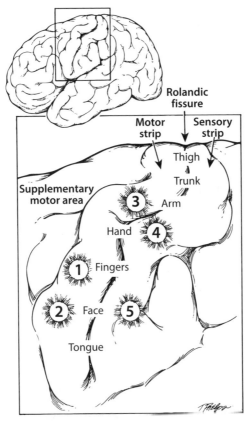

FIGURE 2.3. Motor and sensory areas of the brain. Electrical stimulation at area 1 causes twitching of a finger; at 2, facial movements; at 3, jerking of the arm; at 4 in the sensory strip, tingling in the hand; at 5, tingling of face or lips.

in area 4, then the patient may experience a tingling or funny feeling in the hand (on the opposite side of the body); if the seizure begins at area 5, then the feeling might be in the face or lip.

Focal motor or focal sensory seizures such as these do occur. Michiko's seizures (see the beginning of this chapter) are focal motor seizures involving the lip and face, occasionally spreading locally to involve one side of her face. Seizures may start locally, then spread slowly or rapidly to include other areas of the brain. When a focal seizure spreads to other parts of the brain, the initial movement or sensation is the aura, or warning, of bigger things to come.

The Temporal Lobes: Lateral (Outer)

The outside of the left temporal lobe is involved in aspects of speech. Someone with a problem in one of these areas may have difficulty finding the correct word to use; the person may know the correct word and yet be unable to say it, or may be able to say words (or repeat words) but not be able to say them clearly, or may be able to talk clearly and fluently but not make sense. These are all called *expressive* problems, difficulties in verbally expressing thoughts. The type of expressive problem depends on exactly which part of the speech area is involved (Figure 2.4). Abnormalities in other, slightly different areas of the temporal lobe may cause *receptive* problems, an inability to understand words or phrases, difficulties in language comprehension.

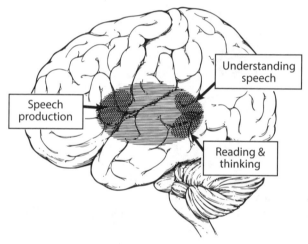

FIGURE 2.4. Speech and language areas of the brain. Areas in the temporal (and frontal) lobe, usually on the left side, are responsible for speech and language. Specific functions appear to lie in relatively discrete areas on the outside of the brain.

Stimulation of the left temporal cortex with small amounts of electricity can locate precisely which part of the brain is involved in each function and can simulate these difficulties. Problems in finding or saying words also occur during or following focal seizures and thus can often aid the physician in identifying where the seizure began or propagated (moved). There is no comparable localization on the outside of the right temporal lobe except in *some* left-handed individuals.

The Temporal Lobes: Mesial (Inner)

The mesial, or middle, inner aspect of both temporal lobes is of great importance in epilepsy, since they are quite prone to damage and are frequently the source of seizures. (This area of the brain and some of its features are shown in Figure 2.5.)

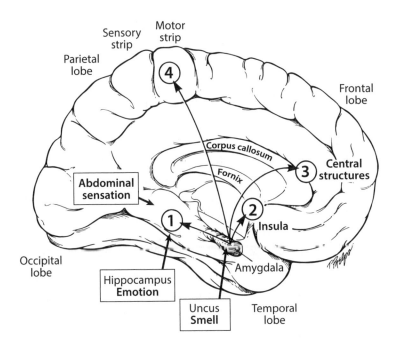

Figure 2.5. Temporal lobe, inner side, and spread of seizures. The inner side of the lobe is often involved in seizures. Change in functions during a seizure can indicate the location of the electrical discharge. The amygdala, hippocampus, and uncus are among the most important of these areas. With their many interconnections to the frontal lobe, they influence emotions, consciousness, and autonomic function. If a seizure starts in the uncus, the aura may be an unpleasant smell. It may then spread to the hippocampus (1), followed by a sensation of fear, or to the insula (2), causing abdominal sensation, then spread to other central structures (3), causing loss of awareness and a complex partial seizure, or to the motor area (4), causing a tonic-clonic seizure.

Stimulation of the front of the mesial temporal lobe, or seizures originating from that part, may produce a smell, usually an unpleasant, acrid smell, often described as the smell of burning rubber. Stimulation farther back in the mesial temporal lobe may produce abnormalities of taste (bitter, metallic) or sensation in the abdomen (cramps, discomfort), or a rising sensation from the abdomen to the throat (as if nauseated).

Also in the mesial part of the temporal lobe are structures called the amygdala and hippocampus, important structures connected to areas of the brain involved with emotions, such as fear, and controlling functions such as blood pressure, heart rate, and paleness or facial flushing (autonomic functions). Billy's seizure began with the sensation of fear, probably originating in this part of his brain and spreading to involve autonomic functions (the pale skin color he displayed) before becoming generalized and spreading throughout the brain. This part of the brain is also involved in storing memories. Thus, stimulation (or seizures) may produce flashbacks, memories, or feelings, as if something had been seen or experienced previously (*déjà vu*). Electrical stimulation of these areas, or spontaneous electrical activity such as seizures, may create or re-create one, all, or any combination of these feelings and experiences.

Seizures that begin in the temporal lobes may remain focal or may spread slowly or rapidly. For example, seizures starting in the uncus (see Figure 2.5) may initially consist of just a peculiar smell (such as burning rubber). This may be the only thing that happens during a seizure, or the seizure may spread to the hippocampus (1) and be followed by a sensation of fear (amygdala). The spread may be to the insula (2) and cause a choking sensation, or a rising sensation in the abdomen and chest or abdominal discomfort. Further spread to area 3 may lead to loss of awareness, with staring, often accompanied by automatic, unconsciously repeated movements, such as lip smacking, picking at one's clothes, and wandering around aimless and confused. These movements are called automatisms. Spread of the seizure from the uncus (1) to the motor strip (4) may lead to a focal motor seizure, a seizure affecting one side of the body (unilateral seizure), or a seizure spreading throughout the brain (a generalized seizure).

Because so many diverse functions are either in or closely connected to the temporal lobe, seizures coming from this area can have various manifestations and may alter consciousness.

Consciousness, or awareness, is not located in any single area of the brain. A surgeon can remove half of the brain (either half), and consciousness remains intact. Loss of consciousness is experienced when either both sides of the cortex malfunction simultaneously or when there is an interruption of the communication between the cortex and the more centrally located deep parts of the brain. Alterations in consciousness can be seen naturally during sleep, when the electrical activity of the cortex changes. During seizures that involve alterations in consciousness, the electrical activity of the cortex as a whole or deeper brainstem connections are always altered.

The Frontal Lobes

Areas of the frontal lobes other than the motor strip are less well defined; they are responsible for personality, memory, anxiety, alertness, and awareness. Because there are so many major connections between the frontal and temporal lobes (see Figure 2.5), it is often difficult to determine from the way a seizure looks whether the function being disrupted is in the frontal or the temporal lobe. Some areas in the supplementary motor area, near the motor strip (see Figure 2.3), seem to control the coordination of movements of groups of muscles. Electrical stimulation of, or seizures in, the supplementary motor area thus may cause the eyes, head, and body to turn away from that side and may appear to cause brief staring and loss of awareness before some of the stereotypical seizures, called focal impaired awareness seizures, appear (and as mentioned previously, these can also come from the temporal lobe).

Other Areas of the Brain: The Occipital and Parietal Lobes

The occipital and parietal lobes are less common sources of seizures, but they can be the most important areas for some people's seizures. The primary function of the occipital lobe, located in the back of the brain (see Figure 2.6), is vision. Messages from the retina (the back of the eyeball) are transmitted through the optic (eye) nerves along a pathway (optic radiation) to the occipital lobe, where vision is registered by the brain. Objects off to your left side (when you look straight ahead) register on the right side of each retina (Figure 2.6), and the message proceeds along the path to the right side of your brain. Images of objects on your right (when you look straight ahead) go to the left side of your brain. Vision is complex, and when one stimulates the occipital cortex electrically, the patient sees only bright lights in a random pattern. When a seizure begins in the occipital lobe—which is not common—flashing bright lights may be experienced off to the left side if it occurs in the right cortex, or to the right side if the left cortex is involved.

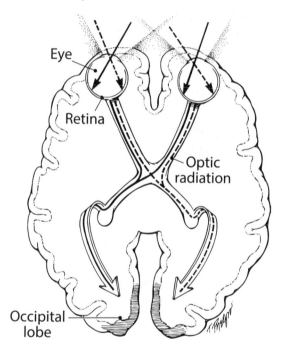

Figure 2.6. Occipital lobe and visual pathways. Vision is located in this lobe. An image on a person's right side is seen by the left portion of the retina in each eye (solid line); electrical impulses from the left side of the retina travel through the visual pathways to the occipital lobe of the cortex on the left side.

The parietal lobe is where perception comes together, where much of what we sense by vision or touch achieves meaning. Here, those flashing lights become patterns forming a visual image; through interconnections with the frontal lobe (where memories are stored), we are able to store the images as memories or to recall formed images as recognized faces or scenes. The posterior temporal-parietal lobe is the site where sounds heard become the pattern of words, which are recognized and remembered or given meaning by association with prior experiences stored in the frontal lobes. It is where speech that is heard becomes speech that is understood and where the sense of touch and feel of a particular object is identified as a key, a ball, or a block. Thus, the parietal lobe is called the *association cortex*. It is rarely the source of seizures and seems to play little role in our understanding of the types of epilepsy. It is not, in other words, very epileptogenic.

This basic and simplified lesson in brain anatomy should provide a better understanding of the many variations of focal seizures discussed below.

Focal Onset Seizures

Motor Onset

Seizures may start with motor involvement of the limbs or parts of the face. These may appear as chewing or picking at clothes (automatisms), loss of tone or posture (atonic), jerking (clonic), brief but sudden trunk bending with either flexion or extension of the limbs (epileptic spasms), vigorous movement of the limbs (hyperkinetic), lightning-fast individual jerks (myoclonic), or stiffening (tonic).

Nonmotor Onset

Because a seizure may begin in areas of the brain that control involuntary functions (see Figure 2.5), it may start with the face becoming pale or flushed. The heart may begin to beat rapidly; there may be abdominal cramps and discomfort or a fullness in the chest or throat. Physicians call these *autonomic* symptoms because the autonomic part of the nervous system regulates involuntary body functions like heart rate, blood pressure, and bowel function. Since the autonomic system has to control both sides of the body simultaneously, not a single half at a time, the physician often cannot identify the side of the origin of the seizure by these manifestations alone.

Seizures can also start with cessation of ongoing behavior (behavior arrest)—continuous movements and interaction stop midstream (children may stop an ongoing task or stop talking midsentence). This type of seizure can be caused by either focal or generalized seizures (see below), so this finding is not specific to focal onset seizures. Seizures can cause problems with thinking (cognitive), with the interruption of skills like using language or doing math.

One of the more difficult to understand types of seizures starts in parts of the brain that either trigger or stimulate emotions or stimulate the recall of prior experiences (emotional). Fear is one emotion frequently experienced alone or as the aura of a seizure, as in Billy's case. The emotion is often described in vague language: "I just felt scared." "I can't describe it—it's a weird feeling." "I know something's going to happen; I know it's coming." A child may not be able to describe the feeling at all, but their face may look frightened, and they may run to a parent and hold on tightly. But, occasionally, feelings expressed are more specific. A scene experienced in the past will be reexperienced spontaneously; voices will be heard, though often they cannot be understood. (These feelings must be carefully differentiated from the hallucination of drugs or psychiatric illness.) Occasionally a person will have the sensation of *déjà vu*, that they have experienced something before (even if it has not previously occurred) or that they have seen someone before; or they might experience *jamais vu* (never seen), in which something or someone familiar seems to be unknown.

Similar experiences may have occurred to each of us on occasion. But when they recur, are frequent, are stereotyped, or are associated with other episodic changes in function or behavior, they may be focal aware seizures.

Finally, different types of sensations can indicate the start of a (sensory) seizure. Examples might include tingling, pain (like electricity), smells (especially something burning), tastes (typically, metallic), visual phenomena (seeing spots, colors, or lights), sounds, or movement (vertigo).

The location of the jerking or sensation on the body depends on where in the brain the electrical activity begins and how it spreads. Since motor and sensory functions are lateralized—one side of the brain controlling the other side of the body—the motor jerking or sensory feeling will be one sided, on the side opposite the brain's activity. Focal seizures may stay local or spread slowly up or down the motor strip or the sensory strip (see Figures 2.1 and 2.2) in a slow spread, or "march," that used to be called a Jacksonian seizure.

Olga comes running to her mother. "I've got that feeling in my hand again. I think I'm going to have another seizure." In a few moments, she develops jerking of the arm and then of the whole side of her body. What kind of seizure is this? Where did it start in the brain? Would it have been a different kind of seizure if it had begun with jerking in the hand or foot or with autonomic or psychic symptoms?

All such events are focal aware seizures starting in one of several areas of the brain. They may or may not spread to involve other brain areas.

Level of Awareness during Seizures

Some seizures, known as focal aware seizures, do not have an alteration in awareness at their onset. Children can have a regular conversation while the seizure is happening—while a limb is twitching or they are having a strange sensation. It is very important to identify this type of seizure because it gives us a clue as to where the seizure is starting, and as they get older, children and adolescents can sometimes describe what they are feeling in a meaningful way. Nonetheless, this is not always the case. Because the functions located in the temporal lobe and in the frontal lobe are complicated, seizures beginning there can be very complex. In addition, many interconnections of both frontal and temporal lobes to other areas of the brain—centrally located—control alertness and awareness. Thus, seizures may alter consciousness. If they do, they are termed *focal impaired awareness seizures.*

A focal aware seizure may spread quickly to the areas that affect consciousness and may result in staring, confusion, loss of alertness, or aimless movements. They are focal aware seizures with a secondary spread sufficiently slow that we can recognize where they started. These seizures are most likely to begin in the temporal lobe (Figure 2.7).

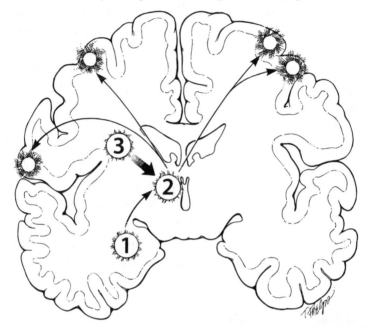

FIGURE 2.7. Examples of spread of focal seizures. If electrical activity remains confined to area 1, there is a focal aware seizure, manifested possibly by sensory, autonomic, or psychic symptoms, all functions located in the temporal lobe. If activity spreads to 2, an area that controls consciousness, alertness, and awareness, cortical function is altered, and the patient stares, is confused, or wanders aimlessly—in a focal impaired awareness seizure. If the spread from 1 to 2 is so rapid that symptoms of the seizure in area 1 are not detected, *or if* the seizure begins at 3 (in the frontal lobe) and spreads to 2, it will produce the same alterations in consciousness. This is also a focal impaired awareness seizure.

Focal impaired awareness seizures may not produce changes in behavior or function before alterations in consciousness occur. Children may start staring blankly without any warning or aura, then wander around the room, pick at their clothes, do repetitive movements, and so on. Such seizures, with sudden impairment of consciousness, are likely to originate in the frontal lobe.

Distinguishing between focal impaired awareness seizures with focal aware onset and focal impaired awareness seizures may be difficult or impossible. It may require careful analysis of a video EEG, showing the instantaneous correlation of changes in the EEG and changes in behavior recorded by the video. The correct differentiation between these two subtypes is not important unless surgery is being considered, but there might be implications for driving in older adolescents and adults.

Sometimes, seizures start in one place (a focal seizure) but then spread to both sides of the brain and look like stiffening and jerking on both sides of the body. The second part of this type of seizure looks like one type of generalized seizure (which is discussed next). These are now known as *focal to bilateral tonic-clonic seizures*.

Generalized Onset Seizures

It seems intuitively obvious that the brain is unlikely to have a seizure all over at one time. A seizure must start somewhere, but in most generalized seizures, the source appears to be on both sides of the brain, very deep in the internal regions. As technology improves, we are finding that some generalized seizures start in an area of abnormal cortex and spread so rapidly that without special techniques, we cannot find the origin. Knowing that a generalized seizure starts in one place and rapidly spreads is important, however, because a source may be identifiable, and the seizures may prove surgically treatable. Without an identified source, surgery is not an option.

Motor Seizures

Tonic-clonic seizures, formerly called *grand mal* seizures, are the sort most people think of when seizures are mentioned, partly because of their portrayal in popular media. The most memorable and frightening type of seizure to the observer, they are the most common seizure type in children, although not in adults.

In a tonic-clonic seizure, the person initially stiffens and simultaneously loses consciousness (and thus is unaware of events). The stiffening is called the tonic phase and causes the individual to fall to the ground. The eyes "roll back in the head," the head goes back, the back arches, and the arms stiffen, as do the legs. This is similar to what happens during a myoclonic, extensor seizure, but this tonic phase of a tonic-clonic seizure happens more slowly. The extension continues for what seems like an eternity but rarely lasts more than 30 seconds.

Because all the muscles contract during this tonic (stiff) phase, the chest wall muscles and diaphragm contract as well, sometimes making it difficult for the person to breathe. They may turn somewhat blue about the lips and face (due as much to the face being flushed with the bluish blood of the veins as to the lack of oxygen). Saliva may cause a gurgling sound in the mouth or throat.

The blueness, gurgling sound, and occasionally tongue biting may cause observers to exclaim, "He swallowed his tongue!" This is a common misconception. A person cannot swallow their tongue because it is attached by a large muscle to the bottom of the mouth and throat. "Quick, stick something in his mouth to keep him from biting his tongue!" someone else may advise, but this is very bad advice. At the onset of the tonic phase of a seizure, the jaw tightly clenches, and attempts to pry it open and put something in may lead to several complications, including biting off the object that was put in the mouth (hopefully not a finger), aspiration of that object, or broken teeth.

After the tonic phase of a tonic-clonic seizure, rhythmic jerking begins. This is the clonic phase. The fists are tightly clenched, the arms repeatedly flex at the elbows and then briefly relax. The legs flex at the hip and knee joint in a similar fashion; the head may flex and then fall backward. These movements are rhythmic and rapid, initially several per second, but then slowing. This rhythmic jerking seems to last forever, although only occasionally does it last more than a few minutes. Then the jerking becomes less severe and occurs at a slower rate, finally ceasing. The end of the jerking is usually accompanied by a deep sigh, after which normal breathing resumes (although because all of the throat muscles are relaxed, there may be a snoring sound with breathing).

The seizure is now over, but the child is not awake and will not yet respond. This postseizure period is the postictal state. In reality, the brain is quite active, but its major activity is to inhibit (stop) the cells from firing. This inhibition has brought the seizures under control.

The postictal period often lasts a few minutes, longer if the tonic-clonic period has been long. If left alone, the person may sleep, but they can be aroused and may feel tired and confused. Muscles may be sore, and the tongue may have been bitten (and bleeding). The best course of action for an observer at this time is to be supportive and reassuring. Allow the person to rest until they are alert and able to go their own way.

A patient may on rare occasions experience a clonic seizure with the rhythmic movements previously described but without the preceding tonic phase. Similarly, a seizure occasionally may be limited to the tonic (stiffening) phase without the shaking. The tonic phase lasts for only a short while, usually less than a minute, and may be followed by a postictal sleep. Management during and after the clonic seizure is identical to that after a tonic-clonic seizure.

There is no important distinction among these last three types of seizures—tonic, clonic, and tonic-clonic—formerly called *grand mal* seizures. Their causes are variable, their outlooks are the same, and their management with medication is identical.

Myoclonic seizures *(myo* meaning "muscle," *clonic* meaning "jerk") are abrupt jerks of muscle groups. A hand may suddenly fling out, a shoulder may shrug, a foot may kick. Occasionally, the entire body may jerk, as in a startle response. *Not all myoclonic jerks are seizures.* Myoclonic jerks can come from the spinal cord, not just from the brain. In fact, they are not always abnormal. While drifting off to sleep, people without any medical problems may suddenly experience a jerk of the body and startle awake. This is a normal phenomenon called *sleep myoclonus* and is *not* a seizure.

An abrupt increase in tone in a muscle group will cause a sudden movement of that part of the body. An abrupt increase in tone in the flexor muscles will cause the body to bend forward at the waist, the head to drop down on the chest, the arms to bend at the elbow, or the knees to come up to the chest. Any or all of these movements may occur during a myoclonic jerk or during myoclonic seizures. If they occur when a child is standing, the child may suddenly be thrown to the ground, perhaps hitting their face, breaking a tooth, or cutting their forehead. If the tone is suddenly increased in the extensor muscles, the head may be thrown back, the back arch, the legs extend, and the arms stiffen. A child who is standing may be thrown backward to the ground.

Myoclonic seizures can be serious, because they may be difficult to control and because they are often only one manifestation of a more involved epilepsy syndrome (see Chapter 8).

Some varieties of jerks and myoclonic seizures are termed *myoclonus of infancy* (or childhood). They can be benign because they are typically outgrown. The term *benign* is often more easily applied in retrospect, but development and school progress should be monitored.

Myoclonic seizures are like being jolted by an electrical shock. They are single jolts. On rare occasions, infants and young children may experience a *series* of these jolts, sometimes even many series per day. Such a series of myoclonic jerks constitutes a special, serious form of epilepsy called *infantile spasms* (see Chapter 8).

Atonic seizures, like myoclonic seizures, are sudden single events. Rather than a sudden increase in tone causing movement of a joint or flexion or extension of the whole body, however, atonic seizures are a sudden *loss* of tone or posture. Arms, legs, or torso muscles, instead of supporting the body by their tone, suddenly go limp. The body slumps or gives way. The arms may suddenly fall, the legs give way, or the body crumple to the ground.

Atonic seizures, like myoclonic seizures, probably originate in areas deep in the brain stem that control muscle tone. Since the areas that increase tone are close to those that decrease tone, children with seizures involving sudden changes in tone may have either myoclonic or atonic seizures and often both.

Nonmotor (Absence) Seizures

An absence seizure, formerly called *petit mal,* is a special and uncommon type of seizure. It starts suddenly and without warning. The child displays a glazed look and stares. They do not know what is happening and usually cannot later recall things that occurred during the seizure. Occasionally, there is a little eye blinking, head bobbing, or mild twitching. The episode usually lasts just seconds, occasionally as long as 15 seconds, and ends just as abruptly as it started. When the seizure ends, the child is immediately alert and back to baseline. There is no confusion afterward. These seizures may occur many (up to hundreds of) times a day and are often mistaken for daydreaming (in fact, this is one of the most common reasons children are referred for evaluation).

It is usually easy to produce an absence seizure in the office by making such a child take deep breaths (this should only be done by a trained professional in the office, not at home). Usually 15 to 30 deep breaths (hyperventilation) will produce a typical spell. (Surprisingly, exercise, such as running, swimming, or bike riding, which may make someone out of breath, does *not* produce one of these spells.)

A parent may see only a few seizures because the brain's activity must be interrupted for more than two to four seconds before a spell is apparent. Thus, very brief electrical events (less than one second in duration) are observable only on the EEG. But, in a sense, the child's awareness may be interrupted frequently, and the child may miss some of what is going on around them.

Occasionally a person who has these spells describes life as being "like a movie from which brief segments have been cut out." Teachers describe the child as daydreaming (and in fact, there may be academic problems because of repeated missed segments of instruction). Friends may call the child "spacey."

Atypical absence seizures are similar to absence seizures but may have more pronounced motor symptoms, such as tonic or clonic spells, or may have automatisms (involuntary behaviors) as seen in focal seizures. They also are less frequent or more prolonged than more typical absence seizures. Atypical absence seizures are more commonly seen in children with neurological illnesses and are often associated with other types of seizures.

Differentiating between Types of Seizures

One of the most confusing areas of classification for both physicians and parents is differentiation between absence seizures and focal impaired awareness seizures. This differentiation may be important, because it may determine which medications should be used to treat your child.

Further confusion comes when trying to differentiate either of these staring spells from normal daydreaming. Let us give you an example of how we try to differentiate daydreaming from seizures.

The teacher called to say that Lisa is daydreaming in school. You have noticed some episodes of "daydreaming" at the dinner table. Does she have absence seizures? Does she have atypical absence seizures? Does she have focal impaired awareness seizures, or is she daydreaming?

The questions your child's physician will want to ask you about Lisa are:

• How frequently is she having these episodes? Daydreaming would occur infrequently and be situational. Absence seizures may occur many times a day. Focal impaired awareness seizures rarely occur more than several times a day or week.

• How do these episodes begin? While most seizures have an abrupt onset, occasionally focal impaired awareness seizures begin slowly, and a warning precedes them. Daydreaming usually does not start abruptly.

• Can you interrupt these episodes? Daydreaming can easily be interrupted by calling the child's name or by physically touching them. Seizures, on the other hand, cannot be interrupted.

• How long does the episode last? Daydreaming can go on until something else catches a child's attention. Absence seizures rarely last more than 15 seconds. Focal impaired awareness seizures may last up to several minutes.

• What does the child do during the episode? While daydreaming or during absence seizures, children are likely to stare into space. During focal impaired awareness seizures, children are likely to smack their lips, pick at their clothes, or display other automatisms.

• What is the child like when she comes back? The child who is daydreaming or having an absence seizure will be immediately alert. The child with a focal impaired awareness seizure will usually be confused for seconds or minutes.

• Does the child remember what was said during the episode? While daydreaming, the child may be aware of what is happening but not pay attention. During a seizure, the child is not fully aware of what is happening around them.

• Do the spells occur only at certain times? If they happen only, say, in math or geography class, the child is likely to be daydreaming. If they occur at random times or whenever the child is tired, they are more likely to be seizures.

With these careful observations, you and your child's physician can usually differentiate the type of episode.

Locating the Site of Onset

All focal seizures may at times spread to affect the whole brain. This spreading typically results in a tonic-clonic seizure. Depending on the direction of the electrical spread, however, it may result in an atonic seizure, in which a child suddenly collapses to the floor or is thrown down, or a tonic seizure, in which the child suddenly stiffens and arches their back.

The parent should carefully observe the onset of a seizure and its progression so that the physician can have an accurate history to determine if there was focal onset, aura, or warning. As with focal seizures, a focal onset of a bilateral tonic-clonic seizure implies a focal problem or disturbance. Bilateral tonic-clonic seizures with focal onset require an especially careful medical evaluation, because if these seizures are not controlled with medication, and if the focus can be identified, there may be a possible cure of the seizures by surgical removal of the area where the seizure begins.

Now, with some understanding of the brain's anatomy, organization, and function, you should be better able to understand the many kinds of seizures and the different names physicians use when they describe your child's seizure or seizures. This naming is important because it will help determine the treatment for your child.

PART II

Diagnosing Seizures AND Epilepsy

CHAPTER 3

How Doctors Diagnose a Seizure and Decide What It Means for Your Child

Was It a Seizure?

A seizure, as we have seen (Chapter 1), is a sudden change in behavior or in motor function caused by an electrical discharge in the brain. A seizure seems easy to diagnose, since it is simply a sudden change in behavior or motor function. But sometimes it's not that simple; children can have sudden changes in behavior for several reasons. Sometimes children faint, daydream, or fall down. How do you tell if those events are seizures?

The only way to diagnose a seizure is to take a careful history of the event that has occurred. That is why doctors ask all those questions: What was the child doing when it happened? What was the first thing that was noticed? What happened next? What was the child doing during the episode? The doctor may ask you to demonstrate what you saw (if you saw it). Was the child trembling, making rapid movements of the arms or legs, or were the child's arms or legs jerking rhythmically? What was the position of the child's eyes—were they open, fixed in one direction, or closed? What was the child like afterward? Were they tired? Did they have a headache? Did the child wet/soil themselves during the spell? While none of these findings is specific for a seizure, the pattern may make the physician more or less suspicious that the episode was a seizure.

There is no diagnostic test for a seizure or for epilepsy. The diagnosis rests solely on the physician's interpretation of the history of the episode that occurred. Although many persons with seizures and epilepsy have abnormal encephalograms (EEGs), many do not. EEGs do not tell the whole story. At times, the EEG may need to be repeated. Some children without seizures may have abnormal EEGs. Changes in an EEG in the absence of change in a person's function are not necessarily seizures that need to be treated themselves but may provide information about risk of seizures at other times.

Since physicians rarely have the opportunity to see the seizure events for themselves, they must depend on the observation of those who witnessed the episode. Most of the time, observers are upset and panicked by what they have seen. On occasion, the physician may ask the observer to enact the event to get a better idea of what happened. Ideally the history should be obtained directly from the person who witnessed the event, but that may not always be possible. Frequently, events occur at school or when the child is with friends. This is one of the reasons that you as a parent are such an important member of the team. You may need to talk to teachers, friends, or even other children who saw what happened. The physician cannot make a diagnosis without good information.

Let us give you an example of how difficult it may be to determine whether a particular episode was a seizure and how we think about the episode's importance for the child's future.

Jane is 13 years old. A nurse is cleaning her arm with alcohol in preparation for taking blood tests ordered by her physician. The nurse takes out the syringe and needle, and Jane says, "Wait a minute, I don't feel well." She looks pale and sweaty, then collapses in the chair. She stiffens and has jerking of her arms and legs that lasts perhaps a minute. Was that a seizure? "Yes," the physician says, "but it was a seizure due to fainting. That is what is called 'convulsive syncope.' Jane fainted, just as many people faint when blood is taken. In some people, fainting is enough to trigger a brief seizure. It's nothing to worry about. That is not epilepsy. She'll be fine."

That diagnosis was easy. Jane's seizure occurred because of fainting. The episode was witnessed from the start by people trained to observe carefully. They heard Jane say she didn't feel well. They saw her become pale and sweaty before losing consciousness. It was clear to them that

Jane had fainted and then had a seizure. The episode occurred in a situation in which fainting is common. But suppose Jane had been sitting in the hot sun with her friends at a baseball game when the episode occurred? Could she have been drinking beer or taking drugs? Would her friends have noted the pallor and sweating before she fainted, became stiff, and had the brief jerking movements? If they hadn't noticed the fainting and had seen only the jerking, her doctor might not have known why the seizure occurred and would have been concerned that it might recur. The physician could not have been as confident in saying that it was convulsive syncope.

Even if a single episode was a seizure, it may not require treatment, since most single seizures do not recur. If episodes are recurring, it should not take long for careful observation to determine their true nature. With easy availability of cameras on mobile phones, the best option would be to capture a video of the event. That is easy to say in hindsight but also an important reminder of what to do if another unusual episode happens. Rare episodes will either disappear as mysteriously as they appeared, or they will become sufficiently obvious and frequent to allow proper diagnosis.

Many children have been treated with medication for a seizure all because of incorrect interpretation of a single event, such as fainting. When in doubt about an event or about the circumstances of it, it is usually better to wait and see if a similar event occurs. It is better to live with uncertainty than to allow yourself or your child's physician to be too eager to label the event and begin treatment. If there is doubt about the nature of the event or events, you should explore this further with your child's doctor, whether or not your child is on medication. Even when your child clearly has had a seizure, different seizures will have different meanings for the child's future. The meaning and decisions about evaluation and treatment may depend on the circumstances in which the seizure or seizures occurred.

Provoked and Unprovoked Seizures

Your child is playing outside when his friend comes banging at the door. "Come quick!" the friend shouts. "Something's happened to Mateo!" You

run and find him on the edge of the playground making gurgling sounds
and with his arms and legs jerking. "Was that a seizure?" you ask your
child's physician later. "It certainly sounds like one," she replies. "We have
to be concerned that Mateo might have another one. If he does, then he has
epilepsy—by definition." If by talking to Mateo's friend, his mother learns
that Mateo was climbing a tree, fell, and hit his head, the doctor might
answer differently: "I think he had a slight concussion and a brief seizure,
what we call a 'posttraumatic seizure.' These brief seizures after a child hits
his head are not uncommon and rarely recur. I think that this is what we
call a provoked seizure. I don't believe he has epilepsy or will have epilepsy."

It is not the mere occurrence of a seizure but also the circumstances
under which the seizure occurs that determine if a child is likely to have
more seizures. Furthermore, except in certain situations, children usually must have two or more seizures to say that they have epilepsy.

If a child has several seizures during an episode of meningitis, after a
head injury, with diarrhea and dehydration, or with other acute conditions, these seizures are termed *provoked* seizures, or *symptomatic* seizures, ones that have a defined cause. Just as Jane's seizure after fainting
was a provoked seizure, so was Mateo's after hitting his head. Once the
acute brain disturbance that caused the seizure has resolved, the seizure
should not recur. It is important to keep in mind that acute conditions
such as a head injury or meningitis can cause permanent damage to the
brain, and that damage can later lead to *unprovoked* recurrent seizures
or epilepsy. Permanent damage followed later by epilepsy, however, is
not a consequence of acute symptomatic seizures in children.

Episodes Often Mistaken for Seizures

Many changes in motor function or behavior are commonly mistaken
for seizures. These include fainting, tics and other sudden jerking movements, breath-holding spells, migraine headaches, and episodic changes
in behavior. Doctors who are aware of these types of behaviors can take
a careful history and usually separate them from seizures.

Is It Fainting or a Seizure?

It had been a long church service, and as usual, Isabella had almost been
late. Her alarm had not gone off, and when her mother had called her,

she had barely had time to get dressed. No time for breakfast. Her mother told the doctor, "The sermon was long and dull, and Isabella remembers standing for the hymns and feeling dizzy. The next thing she remembers is waking up outside the church. She doesn't remember passing out. The paramedic who happened to have been there asked me if Isabella had epilepsy. Does she? You'll tell me the truth, Doctor, won't you?"

Fainting spells are commonly misdiagnosed as seizures. Indeed, some people have been treated for "epilepsy" for years when they had simply fainted. Fainting is caused by insufficient blood going to the brain. Since one of the brain's important activities is to maintain consciousness and posture, when the brain does not get enough blood, the person may become dizzy and slump to the floor. This decrease of blood flow to the brain may be due to slowing of, or even brief pauses in, the heartbeat. Or it may result from prolonged standing, the blood becoming pooled in the legs or in the abdomen with not enough blood available to pump to the brain. Or it could result from anemia, insufficient red blood cells to carry oxygen to the brain.

In each case, the lack of blood initially causes pallor, followed by sweating. The child feels lightheaded, or dizzy. The room seems to spin, or darkness seems to descend in front of their eyes, and they slump (not crash) to the ground. As soon as the child is lying down, the heart does not have to pump blood up to the head, the blood supply to the brain is immediately increased, and within seconds they regain consciousness. They will usually still be pale and sweaty, may briefly be confused, and may still feel weak. Even though this child has had a change in motor function and consciousness, they have not had a seizure, since that change was not caused by abnormal electrical activity in the brain.

Fainting can precede and cause a seizure, as in Jane's case, or occur without a seizure, as we have seen in Isabella's story. Fainting spells may occur when someone has gone too long without eating, after giving blood, or occasionally because of insufficient sleep or extreme tension or anxiety or overventilation due to anxiety. In individuals who have low blood pressure, fainting can be brought on by standing up suddenly. One often unrecognized cause of fainting is lack of salt.

Esmira was a long-distance runner. At 15 she led the cross-country championship team. She was running at least five miles a day until the day she passed out in the shower. Because Esmira's sister had epilepsy, her mother was sure that she had had a seizure. When seen by her physician, Esmira was very thin. Her exam was normal except for her pulse, which was a runner's, 55 beats per minute, and her blood pressure was quite low, at 90 over 65. Instead of ordering an MRI and an EEG, her physician asked about her eating habits. Because of her father's high blood pressure, the family added no salt to their cooking, and Esmira avoided salt. She was salt depleted, and the hot shower had caused her blood pressure to drop further. After adding salt to her diet, Esmira felt better, her blood pressure registered 110 over 80 at her follow-up examination, and she had no more episodes of fainting.

When we understand the circumstances and the sequence of events, we should be able to distinguish easily between convulsive syncope (seizures with fainting) and other seizures. The preceding paleness and sweatiness described are typical of fainting but not of seizures. Wetting oneself is more common during seizures than after fainting but can occur in both situations. A child who bites their tongue may be having a seizure, but someone who faints usually does not bite their tongue. If the eyes are open and the child has a fixed gaze, the probability of a seizure is high.

When the sequence of events is unclear, the physician will probably want to wait before making a diagnosis, since it is better to be uncertain than to label the event a seizure. If the child continues to have these episodes, either the nature of the spells will become clear or further tests will be indicated to determine the appropriate diagnosis and treatment. An EEG does not differentiate between fainting and seizures unless an episode occurs when the EEG is running.

Fainting spells are not considered seizures unless they are accompanied by stiffening or jerking. If they are accompanied by stiffening or jerking, they are considered provoked seizures but are not considered serious, since they are unlikely to recur except in similar circumstances. They are not considered epilepsy and do not respond to medications used to treat epilepsy. This convulsive syncope, or convulsive fainting, has no more meaning than the fainting episode itself.

Is It Daydreaming or a Seizure?

"Phillip has become forgetful," you tell your child's doctor. "The other day we were cleaning up the yard, and I asked him to pick up a pile of leaves. He just went on raking up the leaves. I shouted at him a second time, but he ignored me. I got mad, but when I went over to him, he claimed he hadn't even heard me. He seems to be doing that a lot lately."

"It could be a lot of things," the physician replies. "As you know, adolescents often have selective hearing. It could be that he had earbuds in, or was daydreaming or just tired of being nagged. Could he be taking drugs? Since you say that he has been having a lot of these episodes, I suppose that they could be seizures, the kind we call absence, or what used to be called petit mal. Let me get him to over-breathe (hyperventilate) a little bit and see if we can produce a spell."

A teacher may describe a child as "daydreaming a lot" or as "not paying attention." Or, on occasion, a child may report that they are missing short segments of their lessons or brief parts of a TV program or video game. Without seeing a staring spell, it will be difficult to interpret such brief events. Such spells can often be precipitated by hyperventilation in the physician's office; if an episode can be made to occur, physicians can see the spell and interpret for themselves.

Daydreaming can be difficult to differentiate from the brief lapses in attention caused by absence seizures. But daydreaming is common in situations that are boring or when a child is tired, whereas absence seizures can occur at any time. Absence seizures may be seen at mealtimes and interrupt a conversation or eating, situations in which a child is unlikely to daydream. Daydreaming can usually be interrupted by calling the child's name or touching the child. Absence seizures cannot be interrupted. If there are frequent spells, it is helpful to take a home video and discuss it with your child's physician.

Tics

"Charley started these funny movements a couple of weeks ago, Doctor. It's just in his face. He sort of makes these funny faces, not all the time, but they're getting more frequent. I've yelled at him to stop. They drive me

crazy. He'll stop for a little while and then do it again. Now he's started jerking his shoulder and grunting. Do you think he's getting epilepsy?"

Tics, like seizures, are sudden paroxysmal movements. They are usually quicker movements than seizures themselves. While they most commonly affect the head and face, they may affect other parts of the body as well. Unlike seizures, they can be voluntarily controlled for periods. Often the child has an urge to have the tics. A tic may be simple, so that the movement looks like a twitch of a muscle or group of muscles, or it may be a complex pattern of movements, but the child remains fully conscious during the movements. Unlike seizures, the recurrent movements are stereotyped. Seizures rarely look exactly the same from episode to episode because of the variations in spread of the electrical activity in the brain. But most tics are reproduced exactly and should, therefore, be easy to identify. Medications can be used to treat severe tics, but they are different from those used to treat seizures.

Myoclonic Jerks

"We were lying down together on the couch, watching TV, and Pete was just dozing off, when suddenly he had this big jerk, like a seizure. His arms and legs went out like he was struck by a jolt of electricity. Then he was awake, like nothing had happened. This is the third one of these I've seen in the past few months. This isn't epilepsy, is it? I'm worried because Pete's uncle has epilepsy."

Myoclonic jerks are sudden movements, usually of an arm, leg, or both arms or legs, often occurring just as an individual is falling asleep. These are called *sleep myoclonus*, and they are common and normal. Myoclonic jerks during waking hours are less common, but unless frequent, they should be of little concern. Frequent myoclonic jerks can be a form of epilepsy (see Chapter 2).

Breath-Holding Spells

"Ava used to be such a good baby, but now she's got 'the terrible twos.' First, she started with temper tantrums, crying when she didn't get her way. Then she began to hold her breath and turn bluish, and I'd just pick her up, and she would settle down. But now something different is happening, and I'm scared. Yesterday she was running and tripped, bumping her

head. She started to cry, then she just held her breath and couldn't breathe. She turned blue, then she became stiff and arched her back and started to jerk all over. I'm sure she had a seizure."

Have you ever noticed that when your child cries hard, they will often exhale, almost lose their breath or seem to hold their breath for a long time before taking another breath? This is normal, even when the delay before the next breath seems interminable. For reasons that are unclear, some children exhale and delay their next breath longer than others and turn blue or stiffen their bodies and arch their backs or even lose consciousness. This is thought to be related to an immature nervous system. This is a *breath-holding spell*—also termed a *cyanotic breath-holding spell*. It usually lasts from 10 to 60 seconds. In a few children, at the end of the breath holding, a seizure may occur with stiffening and occasional jerking. The blood loses some of its oxygen while the child is holding their breath, and that is why they turn blue. With insufficient oxygen, the child loses consciousness. If the lack of oxygen is severe or if the child's seizure threshold is low, a seizure may be provoked.

Breath-holding spells usually start between 6 and 18 months of age and usually occur when a child cries after anger or frustration, such as when a toy is taken away or the child is punished. In such cases, stiffening and jerking are always preceded by crying and breath holding. Seizures seen in epilepsy, on the other hand, are virtually never brought on by such frustration and are never preceded by similar crying. Breath-holding episodes, even when accompanied by seizures, do not need to be treated with antiseizure medicine, and they do not respond to such medication.

Typical breath-holding spells do not usually require any laboratory tests. In some cases, however, anemia has been associated with such spells; hence this may need to be excluded.

If your child is diagnosed with breath-holding spells, your doctor will explain the benign nature of these spells to you and provide reassurance that your child will outgrow them. When the oxygen level drops, the child will automatically start breathing again on their own, and the brain will be protected. While frightening to watch, breath-holding episodes do not result in brain damage.

Sometimes these breath-holding spells can be aborted or prevented by diverting the child's attention. For this purpose, the best course is to learn to ignore the crying, reward the child's good behavior, and not reward the tantrum and breath holding with attention and concern. The spells will probably then decrease in frequency, and the child will outgrow them usually by five years of age, without long-term consequences. In cases with iron deficiency anemia, treatment of the anemia has been shown to reduce the frequency and severity of the spells.

A second, uncommon form of these spells, misnamed *pallid breath-holding spells*, usually occur after minor trauma such as a bump on the head. The child suddenly stops what they have been doing, with minimal or no crying, turn pale, and may fall down. Occasionally the child will arch their back and, rarely, experience jerking movements. Such spells are not preceded by crying, breath holding, or turning blue. They are caused by *vasovagal syncope*, the medical term for fainting. It occurs because of overactivity of the normal reflex that slows the heart rate. If the heartbeat slows sufficiently, not enough blood is pumped to the brain, and the child loses consciousness and stiffens. These pallid breath-holding spells are the infancy and childhood counterpart of fainting when blood is drawn. The slowing of the heart rate can often be reproduced in the physician's office by pressing on the child's closed eye. If a child has an overactive vagal nerve reflex, the physician will hear a dramatic slowing of the heart rate, at times even a brief pause between heartbeats. If an electrocardiogram (EKG) is running at the time, the increasingly longer interval between heart beats can be documented.

Although they are frightening, pallid spells are usually benign and will be outgrown. Only rarely, when the spells are quite frequent, is it necessary to consider treatment. But treatment should not include anti-seizure medications, because these spells are not seizures. The appropriate medications are those that block the action of the vagus nerve and prevent the slowing of the heart. Research is ongoing regarding some medications that may help in reducing breath-holding spells.

Migraine Headaches

"Keeya has been having headaches for a year or more, Doctor, but these past few months they've become more frequent. Now she has one several times a week, and she is missing a lot of school. She says that they are all over her head but mainly start behind her eyes. She has to come home from school and feels sick to her stomach. She usually goes to bed and wants the lights off because they bother her eyes. Sometimes she will throw up, and then she feels better. She sleeps for a few hours and then is fine. She hasn't had any seizures for almost two years now, but the headache is like the ones she sometimes had after her big seizures. Do you think she could have migraine? I used to have migraine attacks when I was young."

Migraine headaches are not uncommon in children, but they often do not resemble adult migraine. In children these headaches usually occur on both sides of the head (bilateral), and only rarely are they one sided (unilateral) or associated with warnings (auras) such as flashing lights or unilateral sensory symptoms. Migraine headaches in children may build up as pounding headaches, with nausea, and sometimes with vomiting. The child usually tries to avoid light, goes to their room, lies down, and goes to sleep. Such headaches typically last for hours. This kind of an attack is not like a seizure, but the episode is sometimes confused with a seizure when the headache component is less severe or when nausea and vomiting are less prominent. Migraine commonly occurs in families, thus there appears to be a genetic predisposition. Longer duration of the episode and nausea suggest migraine. The presence of other seizures may indicate, however, that the headaches are related to a seizure. The headache of the migraine attack and the headache after a seizure can be similar since both are caused by dilation of blood vessels in the brain.

The EEG may be abnormal both in persons with migraine and in those with seizures; therefore, the EEG is an unreliable procedure for deciding which kind of episode has occurred. In some instances, it may not be possible at all to differentiate between migraine headaches and headaches related to seizures. Indeed, as noted, migraine and seizures may coexist. Migraine is more common in those individuals and families with a history of seizures, and seizures are more common in those with a history of migraine. If the doctor thinks these events are more likely to be seizures, they may suggest a trial of antiseizure medication (ASM); a good response to these drugs suggests that the events were, indeed, seizures. If the doctor thinks these are more likely migraine attacks, they may prescribe antimigraine drugs. Again, a good response to this medication will suggest that these are likely migraines. Migraine has been known to respond to some antiseizure medications, but it is doubtful that seizures will respond to medications now used to treat migraine.

Shuddering Attacks

"Jack has started having some weird grimacing and shivering attacks for the last month. He was totally fine until 8 months of age, and other than these attacks that last for a couple of seconds, he is absolutely fine. Could he be having seizures?"

Shuddering attacks are brief attacks of grimacing and shivering in infants that increase with excitement. They can occur several times a day or less frequently. The child continues to play normally after the attacks. They are benign, and no tests are needed. They generally disappear as the child grows older.

Self-Stimulatory Behavior

"Sheila gets some attacks of stiffening and flushing of her face that last for a few minutes. She crosses her legs and gets agitated if we disturb her. What is happening with her?"

Some infants have episodes of self-stimulatory behavior wherein they seem to stiffen, often with crossing of legs and flushing of face. These episodes may last for several minutes and occur when the child is left alone and is not actively engaged in play. They are seen more often in girls than in boys. They are also referred to as infantile gratification or masturbation. They represent a benign phenomenon that is pleasing to the child, and the child doesn't like to be disturbed. No tests are required nor is any treatment needed. Your doctor should provide reassurance that this is a normal developmental process and resolves as the child grows up. Diversion of children's attention toward things they like can be helpful.

Paroxysmal Behavioral Disturbances

"Santiago has been a terror for years now. We've taken him to several psychologists, and we're on our third psychiatrist. Now he's in a residential school for further evaluation. Something has to be done to control these outbursts before he kills someone. They did an EEG, and now they say that this is epilepsy because the EEG is abnormal. I've read about epilepsy, and Santi has never had a seizure. It's just that when someone frustrates him, or does something he doesn't like, he erupts like a volcano. There's no controlling him. He hits and bites and punches. I'm afraid he'll hurt somebody. Gradually he'll calm down and act as if he's sorry. Could this be epilepsy? I almost hope so, since then we'll have medicine to treat him."

Sudden outbursts of bizarre, often aggressive behavior are not uncommon among children with neurodevelopmental disabilities. Psychiatrists often ask their neurology colleagues if such episodes can be seizures. The answer is virtually always no. Studies have shown that aggression that appears to be intentional almost never occurs during a seizure. If a child is restrained or threatened during the confusion that commonly occurs after the seizure, they may react in a combative but random fashion. In this postseizure confused state, children do not mean to fight back or even understand what they are doing.

Episodic behavioral outbursts are almost always precipitated by an event or by frustration. Seizures never are. Seizures may have a postseizure state in which the child is tired or confused. Behavioral outbursts often do not. The EEG is virtually never helpful. An EEG obtained between seizures or behavioral episodes may be either normal or abnormal and, therefore, does not differentiate seizures from behavioral outbursts. Abnormalities on an EEG (see Chapter 7) can be observed in children who never have seizures.

Repeated episodic behavioral changes, in the absence of obvious seizures, are virtually never seizures and, therefore, do not respond to antiseizure medications. Rare patients have confused even the best neurologists. In these cases, trying to capture the episode on video-EEG monitoring (see Chapter 7) may be the only method of ascertaining what is a seizure and what is not. It is worth noting that the same individual may experience behavioral problems as well as seizures.

Nonepileptic Events and Psychogenic Nonepileptic Seizures

Psychological symptoms may cause intentional or subconscious episodic changes in function or in consciousness that are mistaken for seizures but are not, in fact, originating from abnormal electrical activity of the brain, and hence are not seizures. Although they may closely imitate seizures, such nonelectrical episodes are called *psychogenic nonepileptic seizures* (PNES), or nonepileptic events. They used to be called pseudoseizures. This term has appropriately faded away because it implied that the episodes were faked, or "pseudo." These episodes are not any less significant than real seizures; they are just different. They are not imitation seizures to be dismissed. They are not in the child's imagination. They are not to be punished or rewarded. They are the child's unspoken cry for help and should be considered important and addressed with the help of a psychiatrist or psychologist.

"I'm glad we finally got an appointment with you. Leslie's schoolwork is deteriorating, and the medications do not seem to be helping her seizures. Ever since our divorce she has had seizures, and her doctors have tried every combination of medication. Nothing has helped. Every time she spends a weekend at her father's house, she has a seizure. She falls to the ground, flails her legs and arms, and doesn't respond when we shout at her. I know that her EEG is abnormal. Isn't there something you can do to help? Is she a candidate for surgery?"

Does Leslie really have seizures? It's hard to be sure. Your doctor might ask for a more precise description of the "flailing." The doctor might also check to see what abnormalities, if any, appear on the EEG. They might call attention to the fact that the episodes occurred only at Leslie's father's house and began after the divorce. As with seizures, PNES require therapy but therapy that is quite different from that used for epileptic or electrical seizures. Our first approach would be to take a much more careful history of the events that occurred and the circumstances under which they occurred. We would also take a separate history from Leslie.

"Were you taking your medicine at your father's house? Do special things cause these episodes, for example, an argument or a fight?" Depending on our sense of this story, we would try to decide whether these were epileptic seizures or PNES events.

Since Leslie is having problems in school, and since the medications for presumed seizures have been ineffective, we would probably decrease her medication slowly. We would also inquire about symptoms of depression that might be affecting her schoolwork and contributing to PNES. If the episodes continue despite counseling, we would need to observe an episode and the simultaneous electroencephalogram to see if the episode in question is accompanied by electrical discharge from the brain. Video-EEG monitoring can, at times, be crucial in separating true electrical seizures from PNES. An EEG taken during an epileptic seizure will almost always reveal an abnormality. EEG abnormalities found between episodes do not mean that the episodes in question are seizures.

It is important to remember that a child may have epileptic seizures and PNES. Knowing which is which is vital so that medication can be adjusted to control any epileptic seizures and psychological counseling initiated to treat the PNES.

Other nonepileptic events in infants and toddlers include nonepileptic staring, which is usually brief (<30 seconds), and children are usually responsive without crying. There are no automatisms. Some infants may intermittently roll their eyes upward (paroxysmal tonic upgaze) for a few seconds; others may have head tilt, nodding or shaking movements, sometimes with some jerky movements of eyes (spasmus nutans). These last for several seconds and tend to repeat. They start to diminish around the age of 1 year and disappear between the ages of 3 and 6 years. After feeding, some infants have reflux that may manifest as discomfort, with arching of the back that may be mistaken for a seizure (Sandifer syndrome). Whenever parents have any concern regarding weird movements or behavior, they should take a video clip of the episode and show it to their physician.

The Physician's Evaluation

A careful, detailed history should enable the physician to say that an event was or was not a seizure. If neither conclusion is clearly demonstrated, the physician should confess, "I'm not sure what that episode was," but be reassuring.

1. If the episode was not a seizure, it will not require an EEG. Depending on the nature of the episode, it may not require any further evaluation. It should be treated with reassurance and the physician's assessment of what the incident was: fainting, sleep myoclonus, daydreaming.

2. If the episode clearly was a seizure, the physician should be reassuring and point out:
~ The seizure may not significantly affect the child's future and may not need further testing or treatment.
~ Most single seizures in children do not recur.
~ After a single seizure, most children do not require a brain MRI.
~ After a single seizure, most children do not require long-term medication.

3. If the physician is not sure what the episode was, then either:
~ It will recur, in which case careful observation and description and/or capturing the event on video could help the physician establish the nature of the episodes.
~ It will not recur; in which case it was much less significant.

Thus, in most instances, after a single episode, the diagnosis is rarely critical, since regardless of the nature of the episode, the management is similar, including reassurance of child and family and observation of the child. If the episodes recur often, it should not take long to establish their true nature. If they are infrequent and are not interfering with the child's life, they are less significant. Rare episodes will either disappear as mysteriously as they appeared, or they will become sufficiently obvious and frequent to allow for a proper diagnosis.

If the first episode clearly was a seizure, the physician should:

Ask about circumstances, including
~ acute illness
~ duration of episode

Consider possible causes, including
~ fever
~ metabolic factors
~ stroke
~ infection
~ head trauma

Reassure the family that in most cases, seizures do not recur.

If seizure recurs, the physician should:

Get a good history.

Tell the family what to watch for.

Ask about circumstances, including
~ acute illness
~ duration of episode

Consider possible causes, including
~fever
~ metabolic factors
~ stroke
~ infection
~ head trauma

The child who has clearly had a single seizure needs appropriate testing to determine the cause if:

• the child is, or has been, sick; or

• the child has a progressive neurological problem; or

• the child has remaining neurological deficit.

When the child has a seizure out of the blue, without any of the above conditions, then:

- The child does not necessarily need a CT or MRI.

- The child does not necessarily need blood work.

The child who has not had a seizure, or whose episode was unclear, usually does not need testing, for no test will tell you if the event was a seizure or not. Careful observation, watching and waiting, is often the best approach.

The EEG does not diagnose or rule out seizures. Remember:

- Almost 10 percent of all individuals will have a single seizure at some time during their lives, most often in childhood.

- Of those who have a single seizure, 50 to 75 percent will never have another.

For such reasons, it is not necessary for you or your child's physician to be overly worried about the future just because your child has had one episode, even if that episode was a seizure.

CHAPTER 4

How Doctors Evaluate and Think about a First Seizure

Every child with a first seizure or suspected seizure should be seen immediately by a physician to evaluate for a cause that may require urgent treatment. The first thing your physician will want to know is if your child has a fever. The causes of a seizure in a child who has a fever may be quite different from the causes in a child who has none (Table 4.1).

TABLE 4.1. Potential Causes of a First Seizure

With fever

Febrile seizure
Meningitis (viral, bacterial)
Encephalitis (viral)
Unknown (idiopathic)

Without fever

Unknown (idiopathic)
Chemical imbalance (dehydration, excess fluids, calcium, magnesium)
Trauma
Tumor
Vascular malformation, stroke

NOTE: Seventy percent of first seizures in children are of unknown cause. Also, causes vary with the child's age.

Febrile Seizures

The car screeches to a stop at the emergency room entrance. The mother rushes in with a small infant in her arms. "I thought my baby was dying," she sobs. "I was holding him and giving him his bottle, and all of a sudden he felt very warm to me, like he had a fever. Then his eyes rolled back in his head, he got stiff and started to jerk all over. I gave him mouth-to-mouth resuscitation, and then the jerking stopped. We just got in the car and rushed over. He's sleeping now. Is he going to be all right?"

Many first seizures in a child less than 5 years of age will be what are called *febrile seizures*. These are seizures brought on by fever (typically defined as elevated body temperature above 38° Celsius or 100.4° Fahrenheit) in a child older than 6 months and younger than 5 years of age. These are the most common seizures of childhood and occur in 2 to 4 percent of children. Febrile seizures reach their peak at about 18 months and are, in general, outgrown by the time a child is 5 years old. Most febrile seizures will occur on the first day of illness, and in some cases, the seizure may be the first sign that the child is ill. When a young child has a seizure and a fever, it is urgent that they be seen by a physician to be certain that this seizure is not due to meningitis, an infection in or around the brain caused by bacteria or by viruses, or encephalitis, an inflammation within the brain itself that is usually the consequence of a virus. While bacterial meningitis is less common today because of vaccines, it remains a serious medical condition. With modern antibiotics and with early diagnosis, most children with meningitis can recover without disability. Most viral infections of the brain are mild and are not treated with medications, but for the few severe viral encephalitic infections, treatments are being developed.

When the physician sees your child, they will take a careful history and perform a thorough physical and neurological examination. The physician will look for the cause of the fever. This may include examining the child's ears, throat, or looking for infection in the child's urine or blood. Depending on the child's age, clinical history, and exam findings, the physician may consider a lumbar puncture (spinal tap) and brain imaging to assess for meningitis or encephalitis. A spinal tap sounds frightening, but it is a relatively simple and low-risk procedure in children. Most of the time, however, the child who has a first seizure with a fever will not necessarily need special tests or brain scans.

Fever lowers the brain's threshold for seizures (see Chapter 1). Young children have a lower seizure threshold and thus are more prone to a seizure when a rapidly rising fever further reduces this already low threshold. This is the reason that such seizures tend to occur in young children. The threshold gradually increases over the first years of life as the brain becomes more mature, which is why these infants and young children outgrow the tendency to febrile seizures as they grow older. Febrile seizures are very uncommon after age 5 or 6. Certain families tend to be prone to febrile seizures, suggesting a genetic predisposition.

These three factors—the lower threshold of the child, the degree of the fever, and genetic predisposition—in combination may lower the seizure threshold sufficiently to cause a seizure. A higher fever or more rapid rise in fever may be required to induce a seizure in an infant without a family history of seizures; a lower fever in an infant with such a family history may be enough. In an older child, whose threshold is higher, a high fever may be sufficient with a family history of seizures (febrile or afebrile) but insufficient without a family history of seizures.

The first seizure with fever can be terrifying to a parent. Occasionally the seizure may be mild and brief (no more than slight slumping and loss of consciousness, or a rolling of the eyes back in the head), but often there may be stiffening, jerking or convulsions, and loss of consciousness. Nine out of ten febrile seizures last only a few minutes, usually fewer than 15, but even brief seizures seem to last a lifetime to parents who have never seen a seizure before and who believe that their child is choking, swallowing their tongue, or even dying.

What Should You Do during a Seizure?

A child who is having a seizure should be placed on their side and protected from sharp objects.

Tight clothing should be loosened.

Do not try to put anything in your child's mouth—they will not swallow their tongue.

Do not restrain your child's movements.

Remove harmful objects from nearby.

Time the seizure if you can.

Most of these seizures will stop on their own in a few minutes. If a single seizure lasts more than 5 minutes, or if the child has another seizure soon after the first one, call 911. If the child is still having a seizure by the time emergency personnel arrive, they may give your child medication to attempt to stop the seizure promptly and transport the child to the emergency room. We recommend that any child experiencing their first seizure (with or without fever) be evaluated urgently by a physician.

The child does not necessarily have to stay in a hospital just because they have a fever and have had a seizure. The decision about hospitalization is a judgment based on several medical and individual factors and should be made jointly after you have discussed the situation with the child's medical care team. Most children with febrile seizures will recover from the seizure quickly (within an hour) and can usually return home. Children with meningitis or encephalitis may have a varying course—from a mild illness to one that is severe or even life threatening—and probably will need to stay in the hospital for a period.

After the Seizure Is Over

If the seizure has stopped, the physician will want to find the cause of the fever. The most important thing for the physician to determine is whether the child has meningitis or encephalitis. In most cases of febrile seizure, a thorough history and detailed clinical examination may be sufficient to make this assessment. If the child is under 1 year of age, or if there is any concern about meningitis, a spinal tap and/or brain imaging may be performed. Depending on the history and exam, your doctor may recommend other tests to search for the source of the fever that triggered the seizure. In a young child with a first seizure with a fever, however, tests for other causes of the seizure are rarely helpful. If the child has recovered from the seizure and is running around the doctor's office, as is true after most febrile seizures, further testing with scans and EEGs is rarely helpful. The physician can best try to calm your fears by giving you information about seizures of this kind.

Questions You Might Ask

You will likely have many questions about febrile seizures, among them these:

Q. *"Will they have more seizures?"*
A. Only 25 to 30 percent of children who have had one febrile seizure will go on to have another febrile seizure. The risk is increased if the first febrile seizure occurs in the first 18 months of life, occurs in the first hour of an illness with only moderate fever (<38°C or 100.4°F), and if there is a family history of febrile seizure. If the child has none of these risk factors, the chances of recurrence may be as low as 10–20 percent.

A child who has a second febrile seizure, however, has about a 40 percent chance of having a third, and after a third, also a 40 percent chance of having a fourth. But only 9 percent of children with febrile seizures have three or more.

Q. *"The doctor says that since the fever came after the seizure, it wasn't a febrile seizure."*
A. Fever (or illness) can trigger a seizure in someone who has a low threshold (see Chapter 1). A febrile seizure is defined when a seizure occurs within 24 hours of fever. When a child has a first seizure, however, it may not be possible to tell whether it is a febrile seizure or a first nonfebrile seizure merely triggered by the fever. Since neither will be treated—because it was a first seizure—it makes little difference. The chance of another one remains about 25 percent.

Q. *"What will happen if they have another?"*
A. There is no evidence that recurrent febrile seizures damage the brain. Children who have febrile seizures do not develop intellectual disability

as a consequence of the seizures. These children do not develop cerebral palsy as a result of these seizures. There is no evidence that these children have an increased chance of having learning disabilities. Children who have one, two, or even three or more febrile seizures grow up just like children who have never had such seizures.

Q. *"With the first seizure I called 911, and they took Darnell to the emergency room. I was there most of the day while they did the tests. Do I have to call 911 with every seizure?"*
A. No. Calling 911 with the first seizure was the natural thing to do. You didn't know what was happening to your child. Now that you have read this book, you know that most seizures will end on their own. Your child will be fine in a short time. Call for help only if the seizure lasts longer than five minutes, or if your child has back-to-back seizures, or if your child has difficulty breathing after the seizure. Long seizures may require medication to stop the seizure.

Q. *"What about a seizure that lasts more than 30 minutes? Will it recur?"*
A. Only one in ten febrile seizures lasts more than 30 minutes, and most of those prolonged seizures are the initial seizure only. A child who has had a prolonged first febrile seizure is no more likely to have a second seizure than if the first seizure was short. But if the first seizure was long, and the child does have a second seizure, then the second seizure may also be prolonged. For this reason, your child's physician may prescribe a medication such as diazepam (Valium) that can be administered by you at home if the seizure lasts longer than 5 minutes. Intranasal midazolam is also often used to treat prolonged seizures, and physicians sometimes use it in these circumstances.

Q. *"Should medication be given to prevent another seizure?"*
A. Treatment of fever with antifever medications has recently been shown to prevent recurrence of febrile seizures during the same febrile illness course, but it does not seem to prevent recurrence of febrile seizures in future febrile illnesses.

Currently, no medication is recommended to prevent recurrence of febrile seizures. In the past, phenobarbital was often used, but it has potentially significant side effects, such as behavioral changes and an adverse effect on intelligence. Diazepam was often prescribed to be used when a child became ill, but it causes sleepiness and irritability, and one study showed that parents often did not give the medicine in time to prevent another seizure. Either they did not recognize that the child was sick before the seizure occurred, or they did not detect the fever, or the child was at a day care center and the medicine was at home. In short, while diazepam (Valium), if given at the onset of illness, can prevent febrile seizures, it seems to cause more burden on the parents than it relieves. (If a child's first seizure lasted more than 10 to 15 minutes, however, it may be useful to have diazepam, such as Diastat, on hand to use if the child has a second seizure and that seizure lasts more than 10 to 15 minutes. Diastat is an expensive form of rectal diazepam and is convenient and stable even when not refrigerated. For occasional use, it may be preferable to other forms of diazepam.)

With increasing information that the chance of recurrence of seizures is low and the consequences of recurrence few, most physicians do not routinely prescribe these medications, as it is thought that for most children, the risks of medications outweigh the benefits of avoiding another febrile seizure. We consider continuous medication only in the very rare instance of a child who has many seizures with fever, and we rarely use intermittent Valium for prevention of recurrences.

Q. *"What is the chance my child will develop epilepsy?"*
A. Epilepsy is routinely defined as two or more recurrent unprovoked seizures. Febrile seizures do not cause epilepsy. The chance that epilepsy will develop is slightly higher in a child who has had a febrile seizure (1–2 percent) than in one who has not, but not much greater (see Table 4.2). Out of 100 children who have had a febrile seizure, more than 98 will never have epilepsy. The risk factors for epilepsy developing in a child who has had a single febrile seizure are:

- prolonged first febrile seizure (more than 15 minutes)

- one-sided or focal seizure

- two or more seizures during the initial episode

- a family history of epilepsy, especially maternal

- a neurological disorder, such as cerebral palsy, or delayed development before the seizure

- over age 3 when the first febrile seizure occurs

- multiple febrile seizures

TABLE 4.2. Risks Associated with Febrile Seizures

Type of risk	Percentage of risk (%)
Risk of	
Mental retardation	No greater than in
Cerebral palsy	children without
Learning problems	febrile seizures
Death	
Risk of epilepsy	
If there were no febrile seizures	0.5
If there was 1 febrile seizure	2.0
Risk of epilepsy after one febrile seizure with risk factors*	
0 risk factors	1–2
1 risk factor	2.5
2 or more risk factors	5–10

*Risk factors: (1) seizures longer than 15 minutes; (2) two or more on same day; (3) family member with epilepsy; (4) one-sided seizure

A child who has a febrile seizure but none of these risk factors has an approximately 1–2 percent chance of later developing epilepsy. A child with one factor has a 2.5 percent chance, and a child with two or more risk factors has a 5 to 10 percent chance of epilepsy. In rare cases, febrile seizures that last more than 30 minutes may cause scar tissue in the temporal lobe of the brain. In some of these children, epilepsy does develop.

Q. *"Isn't there anything that can be done to reduce even these small risks?"*
A. There is some evidence that having more than ten febrile seizures may increase the chance of epilepsy, as can a first febrile seizure that lasts more than 30 minutes. That is why we always suggest calling for help if a seizure lasts longer than 5 minutes. Nonetheless, there is no evidence that placing your child on preventive medication after a febrile seizure will reduce the risks of later epilepsy. Your doctor may provide a prescription for "rescue medication" to be used if a febrile seizure recurs (see Chapter 11).

Think positively! Your child has a 70 percent chance of not even having a second febrile seizure. Their chances of not developing epilepsy are greater than 90 percent.

Evaluating the Child with a First Seizure without Fever

Now let's talk about the evaluation of a child who has had a first seizure without fever. If your child clearly has had a seizure, your first question, and indeed that of your physician, should be "Why? What caused it?" Since a seizure is the result of a disturbance of normal brain function, and since there can be many different types of disturbances, there are many different causes of seizures (Table 4.3).

One type of disturbance is acute, usually only temporary, and while capable of causing a single (provoked) seizure, it rarely causes recurrent seizures. Since some of these causes—such as infection or trauma— could require urgent treatment, your physician will concentrate on them at the time of your child's first seizure.

Most first seizures without fever are of unknown cause. While not knowing a cause for the seizure is frustrating, the diagnosis of a seizure of unknown cause, often referred to as idiopathic, is the best possible diagnosis for your child. A diagnosis of idiopathic seizure is an occasion for considerable optimism. It means that your doctor hasn't found a serious cause (genetic, structural, metabolic, etc.). More than half of first

TABLE 4.3. Causes of Nonfebrile Seizures

Trauma	*Metabolic conditions*
Birth trauma	Low blood sugar
Head trauma	Low calcium
Tumor	*Infection*
	Meningitis
Structural problems	Encephalitis
Vascular problems	*Idiopathic (of unknown cause)*
Stroke	
Abnormal blood vessels	

Seventy percent of nonfebrile seizures are idiopathic, meaning we don't know the cause. Of all the causes of seizures, these are the most likely type in an otherwise normal child. Idiopathic seizures are also the kind of seizures most likely to respond to medication and to be outgrown.

---

seizures are idiopathic. Idiopathic seizures are likely to be controlled with medication and could be outgrown. If there is a single such seizure, your child does not have epilepsy.

Evaluation of a child who has had a seizure but no fever depends on many factors: the age of the child, the type of seizure, how soon after the seizure the child is seen, and whether the child has returned to normal. The frequency of various causes of seizures changes with the age of the patient. After taking a careful history, the physician will look for general physical abnormalities. Abnormalities of the heart's rhythm or rate, or a significant drop in blood pressure leading to passing out (also called syncope), may lead to a lack of oxygen to the brain; other heart disease may lead to strokes or seizures. High blood pressure can cause seizures, as can acute or chronic kidney disease. Some birthmarks provide evidence of problems in the brain that may cause seizures, so your physician will look carefully at your child's skin. Often, seizures may have an underlying genetic cause. Brain tumors and cancer are rare causes of seizures in children.

Your child's doctor will also want to concentrate on the child's neurological function and on your child's development to detect any new neurological abnormality that might suggest a stroke, infection, or tumor requiring treatment; to verify that there is no abnormality; or to document old neurological abnormalities for comparison with future examinations.

A careful neurological exam does not necessarily require a neurologist. If your child's physician is concerned about some of the findings or discovers suspicious abnormalities, they may want to refer you to a specialist, a pediatric neurologist. If you or your child's doctor simply have concerns about what has happened or what to do, a pediatric neurologist or an appointment at an epilepsy center's first seizure clinic might be helpful. Decisions about testing and treatment do not require the opinion of a pediatric neurologist. Your pediatrician or family physician and this book should help you with your anxiety.

Q. *"You mean that's all there is? You tell us our son has had a seizure, and you're only going to talk to us and examine him. Aren't you going to do any tests?"*
A. There is no laboratory test for a seizure. The diagnosis of a seizure depends on your description of what happened. Some tests can be useful in looking for a cause of the seizure. Certain tests help the physician rule out other peculiar episodes that mimic seizures. The physician may want to do an electrocardiogram if concerned about abnormalities of heart rate or rhythm. They may order blood tests if they suspect diabetes or other chemical problems. But the diagnosis of a seizure itself can be made only by direct observation of the spell by a physician or by their careful interpretation of the observations of others.

As we discussed in Chapter 3, at the end of this detailed history, the physician can say, "That was a seizure" or "That was not a seizure. It was . . . ," or often, "I'm not sure what that was." If the doctor (and you) are certain that it was not a seizure, then usually no further evaluation is necessary. If you and the physician are not certain, then no work-up need be done, either. Wait to see if it happens again. If you and your child's doctor think the event was a seizure, even then no further evaluation may be needed, although usually the physician will order a brain study called an electroencephalogram (EEG) and sometimes an MRI (magnetic resonance imaging). Tests such as EEGs and brain scans do not tell you if it was a seizure.

The most common tests performed when a child has had a possible seizure are an EEG and MRI brain scan. Although an EEG does not diagnose a seizure unless a seizure occurs during the study, it usually offers a perspective, such as the likelihood of further seizures or insight into an epilepsy syndrome and appropriate further evaluation or treatment. An MRI brain scan may, in the proper circumstances, be useful in searching for the cause of the seizure, but a brain scan does not itself diagnose epilepsy. Nor does it rule it out. Although these tests may be useful in determining the cause of a seizure, both EEGs and MRI brain scans can be normal in the child who has had a seizure, or both may be abnormal in a child who has not had and never will have a seizure. A detailed discussion of these tests is in Chapter 7.

In addition, the type of seizure, other neurological abnormalities, or a strong family of history of epilepsy might lead to genetic testing (see Chapter 9). Just as after a first febrile seizure, after a first afebrile seizure you will have many questions: "Will it happen again?" "Can it be prevented?" "What are the risks of prevention?" The remainder of the book addresses these questions for you and will help you get the most appropriate care for your child.

CHAPTER 5

Decision Making

Assessing Risks and Benefits after
a Nonfebrile Seizure

"When are you going to start Frank on medication? What are its side effects?"

"Now that Joyce has had a seizure, how long before I can allow her to ride her bike again?"

"Billy was going to go on a trip out west this summer. Should I put down the deposit? Will he be able to go?"

Life is full of risks and benefits. We take risks for ourselves and for our children every day. Although no one would ever do it, the safest place to raise a child might be in a bubble. In that bubble the child could not be injured when they fell down, tumbled from a tree, or crossed in front of a car. Your child would be safe! But you would be sorry. Clearly, a child raised without risk would be a very abnormal child. Living, therefore, is best seen as a series of assessments of the relative importance of risks and benefits. Making decisions about which risks (costs) to take for which benefits is what we all do subconsciously all the time.

Risk-benefit analysis involves weighing the good against the bad. On the good side of the scale, we calculate the chance and worth of a benefit. A small chance of winning a large amount of money in the lottery may be "worth it" and outweigh the risk involved in losing a small amount of money. Worth has different meanings in different situations and to different people. Achieving "worth" or "winning" always involves some risks and consequences that must be weighed against the potential benefits.

Medicine is a series of risk-benefit analyses. In the past, physicians tended to do all the analysis for you and recommended what you should do—whether your child should take medication and what medications they should take. This approach might be easier for the parent, and perhaps for the provider as well, since it doesn't involve as much time and discussion. With the advent of a more medically sophisticated public, however, the patient and the family are, and should be, more closely involved in the decision-making process. The physician will still weigh the risks and the benefits and make recommendations based on this assessment, but you as parent should weigh them as well. The risks of what the doctor recommends are *your* risks (or your child's), not the physician's, and the benefits that accrue, accrue to *you or your child*. Your evaluation of the worth of the benefits or the consequences of the risks may differ from that of your child's physician.

As we talk about the risks and benefits of the decisions you will now have to make about your child and their seizure management, keep in mind that:

there will be risks and benefits to each decision you make *or don't make*;

these risks and benefits will vary greatly in their consequences and in the magnitude of the consequence, both good and bad;

the risks and benefits are *yours and your child's*, not the physician's; and frequently there are no "correct" or "incorrect" decisions. In many situations, different people will come to different decisions. Whatever decision is made or not made, there are always consequences, and they must be assessed in advance as far as is possible.

No one can accurately predict the future. Consequences are not always foreseeable. Therefore, you and your child's physician must always make the best decision possible without feeling guilty if things don't work out the way you planned.

Whether to Use Medicine

The first decision you face may be whether to treat your child after a first nonfebrile seizure. At one time, physicians believed that a single seizure was the first sign of epilepsy and that a person who had one seizure would inevitably have more. Therefore, after the first seizure, they pre-scribed medication to prevent the recurrence that was "bound" to occur. Today, we, like many other physicians, do not believe this.

We have learned that after a single *convulsive* seizure of unknown cause, the chance of recurrence may range from 20 to 80 percent, de-pending on various factors. Children with a first convulsive seizure and a normal EEG appear to have a low risk of recurrence. Risk is in-creased by the presence of one-sided (focal) seizures, findings of spike discharges on EEG, and existing neurological deficits in the child. Chil-dren with staring spells—absence or focal unaware seizures—are likely to have, or to have had, recurrent seizures. The first seizure of this type rarely comes to the attention of the parent or the physician. The same is also true for myoclonic seizures and infantile spasms.

Q. *"Should my child begin taking daily medication after her first seizure?"*
A. What are the chances that your child will have another seizure? If the chances were 10 to 15 percent, would you consider this a high chance or a low one? The consequences of a second seizure will depend on the child's age and the type of seizure. The consequences of a seizure could be great for older adolescents or adults if, for example, they are driv-ing a car, but the cost of prohibiting driving is also great for this age group. The younger child faces no such concerns. The consequences of everyday activities, therefore, vary with age. The toddler is unlikely to be climbing a large tree, while the older child may be climbing when a seizure occurs. Risks and consequences vary dramatically with age, with activities, and also with personality, as well as many other factors. Since the consequences will happen to you and your child, you (and some-times your child) will have to be the one to evaluate their significance.

Medication is usually started to decrease the chance of another seizure. But does medication do this? Research has found that treatment of the first unprovoked seizure reduces the risk of relapse but does not affect the long-term prognosis of epilepsy. In other words, the chance of long-term seizure remission is not changed by delaying daily antiseizure medication after a first seizure. Yet, treatment with antiseizure medications seems to carry a higher risk of side effects.

You would probably want to try medicine anyway *if* it involved no risks or negative consequences. Unfortunately, there *are* both risks and consequences to medication. Every medication has side effects (risks and consequences). The "cost" in terms of side effects can be substantial. The cost of medication can also be significant for some families, depending on insurance coverage. You have to evaluate the costs and benefits for your child. The seizures can *always* be controlled by enough medication to put your child to sleep. Would that be worthwhile? Think about your child's quality of life when evaluating the risks and consequences of medication.

Q. *"I don't even know the names of the medicines! How do you expect me to know and evaluate the risks of their side effects?"*
A. Ask your child's doctor about the medicines that they might choose if you were to treat. We discuss the various medications and their side effects in detail later in this book. Here is one example of decision making about one medication commonly used in children, levetiracetam. Levetiracetam is a safe antiseizure medicine, but a frequent side effect in children is a negative effect on behavior. Of young children who take this medicine, 12–38 percent may have behavioral issues characterized by agitation, oppositional behavior, aggression, mood lability, and depression. In addition, it may cause psychosis in 2 percent of children and rare cases of suicidal ideation. It can also cause somnolence (sleepiness) in about 15–45 percent of patients, increased blood pressure in 17 percent of young children, rare cases of allergic reactions that can be life threatening, rare cases of serious skin reactions that can be life threatening, and rare cases of blood abnormalities.

To decide whether or not to start levetiracetam, it would be useful to list some pros and cons of the decision. Clearly such a list could be very long, but a helpful list might look something like this:

After a first nonfebrile seizure, if you start your child on levetiracetam, there is

- a chance the child will have another convulsive seizure

- a 12–38 percent chance of behavioral problems developing from the medication, and a 2 percent chance of psychosis as well as a rare chance of suicidal ideation

- a 15–45 percent chance of the child developing somnolence

- a 17 percent chance of a young child developing high blood pressure

- a small chance of a rash developing that will require discontinuing medication, including serious skin reaction

- a small chance of a severe allergic reaction that may be life threatening

If you decide not to start your child on medication, there is

- a 20–80 percent (on average 50 percent) chance of the child having another convulsive seizure

- a zero percent chance of a rash or a severe allergic reaction developing

- a zero percent chance of behavioral problems developing as a consequence of medication

It appears that, after a single seizure, medication reduces the chance of another seizure but does not affect the long-term outcome, and, indeed, levetiracetam, for one, like other anticonvulsant medications, produces its own risks. Are there benefits associated with starting levetiracetam that outweigh the risks?

One benefit of starting the medication may be your sense of security—or false sense of security—that your child will not now have another seizure. Since most children who have had only one seizure will never have another one *whether or not* they are treated, it would be difficult to assess if the use of medication after a first seizure would be responsible for your child's not having another seizure. The use of medication in children who have repeated seizures (epilepsy) can, however, have different and clear benefits.

Each antiseizure medication has its own risks and side effects. Whenever a new medication is considered, you must weigh the risks and benefits of that particular medication.

We at Johns Hopkins usually do not recommend starting every child with a first seizure on medication in part because about half of these children will never have another seizure and in part because there seem to be few consequences from a second seizure. Other physicians may come to different conclusions. Parents may weigh the risks and benefits in different ways. Every child's situation is unique. Therefore, there is no single "correct" answer to the question, "Should we start a child on medication after a first seizure?"

We have discussed the considerations regarding treatment of the child after a first "big" seizure. "Smaller" staring seizures are rarely recognized after only one spell has occurred, and, therefore, they are usually treated when recognized, because we suspect that they are not first seizures but recurrences.

Decisions about Everyday Life

Since you are probably not going to raise your child in a bubble, you will have to assess the risks and benefits of most daily activities with questions like these.

Q. *"Can my child still ride his bike?"*
A. To help you assess the answer, we would have to ask, "How old is your child?" "How frequently do they have seizures?" "Do they have a warning of the seizure?" "How reliably would they respond to that warning?" "How much do they ride their bike?" "How important is bike riding to them?"

You would have to assess how great the chances are of your child being injured on the bike. Any child faces substantial risk of being injured while bike riding. Are the risks much greater after a child has had a single seizure? They have only a 50 percent chance of having another seizure—*ever*. Thinking carefully about your answers to these questions will enable you to be protective, but not overprotective. Perhaps you can be appropriately protective by choosing where they can ride and insisting that they wear a helmet.

Q. *"Can my child swim?"*
A. We were once asked to comment about a lawsuit against a physician who had not prohibited his patient with epilepsy from swimming. The child had drowned, as do a number of children without epilepsy who swim. It was not clear that this child had had a seizure at the time of the drowning. Thinking about whether your child should be allowed to swim involves asking many of the same questions we asked about bike riding. "How old is the child?" "How frequently do they have seizures?" "How important is swimming?" "How well will they be supervised?" *Every* child who swims should be carefully supervised. The child who has seizures should clearly be closely supervised. But, if well supervised, should they be prohibited from swimming? These individualized decisions will depend on your analysis of the risks and benefits. You might wish to consult the American Academy of Pediatrics website for the most current analysis and recommendation about this.

Similar questions can be asked about allowing your child to go out and play, stay at another child's house, climb a tree, go on trips or go to camp, and eventually drive a car.

We permit children without seizures to take risks. We do not want to shelter a child who has seizures from *all* risks. Taking risks is part of the growing process. We want simply to shelter that child from the *increased risk* associated with a seizure recurrence. But this sheltering must be accomplished at an acceptable cost. For children with recurrent seizures, most physicians recommend showers with the door unlocked over bathing. We also strongly recommend use of helmets for riding on anything that has wheels (bikes, scooters, skateboards, ATVs, etc.) and close supervision during swimming. We usually recommend the use of a harness with high climbing. For those with one unprovoked seizure, we recommend practicing these seizure precautions for at least three months.

Assessing risks and benefits remains a personal effort. What is high risk for one person is acceptable to another. The value that one child puts on being allowed to play, ride, or participate in certain activities may be different from the value placed on these activities by their brother, sister, or friend. Physicians tend to be conservative and overprotective. As long as the risks are yours, or your child's, and do not endanger others, then taking them should be your and your child's decision. The physician, the grandparent, or the friend may serve as advisers, but ultimately, they are not the decision makers.

We are frequently asked by parents, "Doctor, what would you do if it were your child? Would you start medication? Would you let them swim? Would you do the surgery?" As we have indicated, each individual gives a different value to the risks and benefits of each decision. "What would you do?" is not a question your child's physician can or should answer.

CHAPTER 6

What to Do during a Second Big Convulsive Seizure

"He almost died!"

"He stopped breathing and turned blue."

"He swallowed his tongue!"

"I almost had a heart attack; I was so upset."

"I just screamed!"

"I called the ambulance, but it took them forever to get here."

"I didn't know what to do!"

Remember, more than two-thirds of children who have one big seizure *never* have another one. If your child does have another, what you should do is stay calm.

"Easy for you to say," you reply. "You've seen a lot of these things. I thought my child was going to die. How can I do nothing? He's my child!"

Certainly, staying calm is the most difficult thing to do. It is easy for the physician or the nurse to recommend, but it's not easy, even for doctors and nurses, to do. Perhaps the most frightening thing about a convulsive seizure is that there is little the observer or parent can do—or should do (see Table 6.1), but understanding some general guidelines may make this less stressful for all involved.

TABLE 6.1. What to Do for a Person Having a Major Seizure

STAY CALM

During the seizure

- Do *not* put anything in the person's mouth.
- Do *not* restrain the person.
- Do *not* call an ambulance (unless the jerking continues for more than 5-10 minutes).
- Do try to lay the person on their side.
- Do put something soft (coat, pillow) under their head.
- Do loosen tight clothing around their neck.
- Do remove sharp objects—chair, table, etc.—from the immediate area.

After the seizure

- Do stay with them until they are awake and alert.
- Do be comforting and reassuring.
- Do allow them to go back to their activities if they are all right.

The stiffness at the start of a "big" tonic-clonic, or convulsive, seizure is called the *tonic phase*. This is when all the body's muscles are contracting together. The child arches their back, and since the muscles of the chest contract as well, the child may let out a scream and then essentially hold their breath. They may turn pale or somewhat blue. This is because the body is protecting vital organs such as the brain and heart and sending less to the skin. In a sense, they *have* stopped breathing, but this phase *will* end. Their heart has not stopped, and you do *not* need to do CPR. Typically, this phase feels like a lifetime, but it is actually only seconds long. When the oxygen gets low enough, the body will usually stop the seizure long before the decreased oxygen can permanently damage brain cells, and the child will breathe normally again.

There is nothing you can do during this tonic phase to get rid of the stiffness or to make your child breathe. Mouth-to-mouth resuscitation will not work, because the muscle contraction will not allow the patient's chest to expand. The most important thing to do is keep them safe from injuring themselves during this period, and if they are not already lying down, lower them to the floor from where they are sitting.

What Should You *Not* Do?

• *Do not* try to put anything in your child's mouth. During the tonic (stiffening) phase of a seizure, the teeth are clenched. If you try to pry them open, you may break a tooth or injure yourself or them. Some people may have heard that a child might swallow their tongue during a seizure. We know that cannot happen, since the tongue is attached to the back of the throat.

• *Do not* try to restrain your child. You cannot stop the rhythmic jerking of the clonic phase. You can place something soft under the child's head to prevent it from hitting a hard surface.

What *Should* You Do?

• You *should* turn the child on their side so that the saliva can run out rather than running back into the windpipe.

• You *should* loosen clothing around the neck so that it does not further impair the child's breathing.

• You *should* clear things from around them, so that during the clonic (jerking) phase of the seizure, the child does not bang themselves against a chair leg or sharp edges of a table.

• You *should*, if possible, put a soft object, such as a pillow, jacket, or shirt, under their head so that their head does not bang against the floor. But don't flex the head downward.

The second phase of a convulsive seizure is the *clonic phase*, in which the muscles jerk rhythmically. Similar to the tonic phase, restraining the child does not help, because the jerks continue anyway. Unless the child is jerking against some sort of hard object, they will not hurt themselves. You *can* gently support the child on the floor, but you cannot stop the jerking. The jerking is not hurting the child; they will not remember it. But it is frustrating for the observer, particularly a parent, to stand by and just watch.

The jerking phase of the seizure usually will last up to several minutes. In an unusual seizure, this clonic phase may last 5 or (rarely) 10 minutes—though it may seem like a lifetime. In general, it is not necessary to call the ambulance unless the tonic-clonic jerking lasts more than 5 minutes by the clock or you are worried about your child for another reason (they hit their head or otherwise injured themselves significantly during the seizure). Generalized tonic-clonic seizures only *seem* to last a long time. Almost all end—by themselves—in 3 to 4 minutes, and typically they are over in under 90 seconds.

When Should You Call for Help or an Ambulance?

Jack was 6 years old and had not had any tonic-clonic seizures for almost a year. His folks had gone out for the evening for the first time in more than a year. Wouldn't you know? Shortly after they left, Jack vomited, felt warm, and started to jerk all over. The babysitter knew that Jack had once had seizures, but she had never seen one. Her first reaction was that he was going to swallow his tongue—if he didn't die first. She called 911. By the time the ambulance arrived, Jack had stopped jerking and was asleep. The emergency medical team listened to his heart, took his blood pressure, and inserted an IV. Within 5 minutes he was on his way to the emergency room.

When told Jack had had a seizure, seeing him still unresponsive, the emergency room physician ordered a CT scan. His examination was negative, but they did not want him to have a seizure in the scanner, so they gave him some lorazepam (Ativan). His CT scan was normal. The blood chemistries showed a little acidosis; he was breathing shallowly, and so they decided to admit him to the intensive care unit and put him on a respirator. Jack fought the intubation and had to be paralyzed. By the next morning, he was fine. The neurologist in the hospital saw Jack and moved him from the intensive care unit, and the following day he was discharged from the hospital.

The sad part about this story is that it happens too frequently. The emergency medical technicians (EMTs) in ambulances are trained to take care of emergencies. A child who has a seizure and is unconscious *might* be an emergency. It is their job to transport that child to the emergency room as quickly and safely as possible. The emergency room physicians are also trained to take care of emergencies. They do not know Jack's prior history of seizure and do not necessarily have the time to evaluate him and his history adequately. A CT scan, while unnecessary in a child who has had a recurrent seizure, could be of value if that child was unconscious for some other reason, like a head injury. Therefore, they ordered the CT scan. The sedation needed to keep a patient quiet during the scan often changes the breathing pattern and, therefore, the blood chemistries. One thing leads to another, and before you know it, this cascade of events lands Jack in the intensive care unit on a respirator.

If anyone had had the time and the inclination to find out the facts, Jack probably did not need an IV, certainly did not need a CT scan, and would not have been intubated or in the hospital at all. It can be hard to stop the cascade of events once 911 is called. This is why we tell parents that unless the jerking is lasting more than 5 minutes by the clock, or there are other concerns, it is not necessary to call 911. Most seizures seem to last forever, but it is a rare seizure that lasts more than 5 minutes and needs medical intervention.

If the Clonic (Jerking) Phase Lasts 5 Minutes, Should You Call an Ambulance?

Virtually *all* seizures will have ceased before this time, and well before the ambulance arrives. The jerking stops by gradually slowing down. Eventually the child relaxes. They often let out a deep breath and then go into a deep sleep. The seizure is over. The brain is recovering. At that point, there is nothing the ambulance crew, physicians, or emergency room personnel need to do but observe.

Why do we say call the ambulance at 5 minutes? Because seizures that last 5 minutes or more are more likely to need a medication to stop them. *If* the clonic seizure is still continuing when the ambulance finally arrives, *then* the ambulance personnel should give an emergency medication to stop the seizure if they can and should take the child to the emergency room. It takes a few minutes to get the child on the stretcher and time to transport them to the emergency room. *If the child is still having a seizure when they reach the hospital, then the emergency room staff may want to give an additional injection to stop the seizure.*

Status epilepticus is a medical emergency and needs treatment. We previously defined this as a generalized tonic-clonic seizure lasting more than 30 minutes (this is discussed at greater length in Chapter 11). This definition was based on the fact that such a seizure *begins* to cause changes in the brain that have the potential for permanent injury. We now know, however, that seizures that don't stop on their own after 5 minutes are not likely to stop without medical interventions. Therefore, we now use an operational definition of status epilepticus as a single seizure lasting 5 minutes or more or back-to-back seizures within a 30-minute period. This definition is intended to guide treatment and ensure that seizures are stopped before the end of that 30-minute period. It does not necessarily imply that there is brain damage when seizures last for 5 minutes or more.

When a typical seizure stops, the child usually lets out a deep sigh and goes into a deep sleep. This is called the postictal period. It is as if the brain is resting from its overexertion. The length of this postictal sleep will vary, depending on the duration and the type of the seizure. It may last anywhere from 10 to 15 minutes up to an hour or two. After a short period, the child can be aroused but often is confused and prefers to go back to sleep. There is no reason not to let them sleep. This sleep is a healthy recovery phase.

On rare occasions, the patient may have a second seizure while still in this sleepy, postictal state. As mentioned above, serial seizures (one after the other without the patient waking up in between) are also termed status epilepticus. When this pattern occurs, the patient should be taken to the emergency room so that these serial seizures can be stopped. They indicate that the brain is irritable and may require medication to de-crease this irritability.

Q. *"Is there anything else I could do during the seizure? Shouldn't I put something in my child's mouth to keep her from biting her tongue?"*
A. The answer is, "No, you should not." Unfortunately, in many gener-alized seizures, children may bite their tongues. But putting something in the mouth is difficult, unlikely to prevent the tongue biting, and may injure them more. Prying the mouth open to put in a spoon or a stick is more likely to break a tooth. *Never put your finger in the person's mouth because it can be badly bitten.*

Q. *"What about mouth-to-mouth resuscitation. Will this help?"*
A. *No!* When the seizure stops, the patient will breathe on their own. During the seizure, your mouth-to-mouth resuscitation cannot get air into the lungs.

It is hard to watch somebody have a seizure and frustrating not to be able to intervene, to stop this terrible thing, not to be able to help. But the best thing you can do is remain calm. By staying calm, you inspire others around you to remain calm; and when your child wakes up, often confused, they will be surrounded by a less anxious, more supportive environment.

Q. *"What about the child who doesn't have tonic-clonic seizures but has seizures where they wander around confused, picking at things, and could injure themselves? What should I do during one of those?"*
A. During this type of seizure, what is called a *focal seizure with im-paired awareness*, the child *is* confused and not really aware of what they are doing or of their environment. They are likely to misunderstand and misinterpret things during this foggy state. If the child is wandering around, try to be protective. The stories about people being aggressive during these seizures come from the child's misunderstanding and mis-interpretation of what is happening and what is being done to them. Seizures that actually cause or present with aggression are very rare. If people try to restrain a child who is in this confused state, they may mis-

understand the motivation and fight back. Rather, you should be protective and reassuring, while trying to direct them away from dangerous objects or from hurting themselves. Take dangerous objects out of their reach and close the door so that they can't wander off. This is perhaps all you can do. Confused ictal and postictal states may last several minutes. Again, only if the seizure lasts more than 5 minutes is it necessary to consider intervention. While these nonconvulsive seizures are less likely to cause injury, the longer they last, the less likely they will stop and the more likely that they will progress to a convulsive seizure and need medication.

Q. *"What happens if my child has a seizure at school or at night?"*
A. Ideally, we could be there with our children and support them through any possible seizures. In reality, a seizure can happen at any time and anywhere. Children with epilepsy who have had many seizures may have specific patterns and triggers that their parents begin to recognize, but the second seizure will often be as much of a surprise as the first. For those that happen at school, educating the child's teacher and the school nurse regarding what the seizure looks like and the seizure first aid discussed above as well as when to and when not to call an ambulance can help your child and the classroom. Schools often have to be extra cautious and will end up calling an ambulance more often than not, but the more comfortable they are, the less likely they will call unnecessarily.

Unfortunately, seizures do occur in sleep. Most parents are concerned about this, worried that they will not recognize that their child has had a seizure. This is always a possibility. Nonetheless, this does not necessarily mean that children who normally sleep alone should be sleeping with parents or under 24-hour surveillance. Some general points may provide reassurance. As mentioned above, the vast majority of seizures stop on their own and do not require treatment. The most violent and longer seizures usually wake up others in the household due to banging or a scream. Even if the seizure is not recognized overnight, children may have symptoms in the morning—a bitten tongue, sore muscles, atypical bed wetting—that lets you know. Some basic precautions in the bedroom may reduce risk of injury, including children not having excessively bulky pillows and blankets that might cover their face, and not sleeping on very high or very soft beds. There are various bed alarms, video monitoring devices, and wearable devices sold commercially that may be able to detect seizures that occur in sleep. Yet, these may also detect non-seizure-related movements, leading to false alarms and, for many families, creating unnecessary stress and loss of sleep. The technology is constantly improving, so the utility of these devices will likely improve over time as well.

Q. *"Can my child die from a second seizure?"*
A. This is, of course, one of the most terrifying outcomes for parents of children with epilepsy or even a single seizure to consider. It is fortunately extremely unlikely, particularly when considering a second seizure in a lifetime, but worthy of discussion regarding epilepsy in general. The fact is that while still rare, the risk of sudden death is increased in people with epilepsy compared to the general population. In addition to cases when injury as a result of a seizure can result in death (such as in a drowning accident), there is a rare phenomenon referred to as *sudden unexpected death in epilepsy*, or SUDEP. As the name implies, this is defined as an unexpected, nontraumatic, and non-drowning-related death in a patient with epilepsy. Specifically, SUDEP is diagnosed when evaluations after death cannot determine a structural or toxic cause. It can be witnessed or unwitnessed, but frequently it is not witnessed. There may or may not be evidence of a seizure, although it is thought to be seizure related, and research is ongoing as to the exact biological mechanisms. What we do know is that those at most risk for SUDEP have frequent seizures and take multiple medications and certain specific medications to control seizures. Those who are at increased risk of SUDEP are also more likely to have generalized tonic-clonic convulsions, certain underlying causes for their epilepsy, a long-standing diagnosis of epilepsy, and a young age of onset. Taking these risk factors together, the child having an unprovoked second lifetime seizure is not at high risk for SUDEP. Whenever a child is given a diagnosis of epilepsy, however, this topic should be discussed between the provider and family.

What Should You Do if Your Child Has a Seizure?

In most cases, support your child though the seizure. Move the things around them to minimize risk of injury. Time the seizure. If it is a convulsive seizure, turn them on their side and make sure that their head is not hitting anything hard. If a convulsive seizure lasts 5 minutes, it is appropriate to call the ambulance.

If the seizure stops on its own and your child returns to their baseline state after a brief postictal state, your child does not necessarily need an ambulance or emergency care unless there are other concerns. In all cases it is appropriate to let your child's physician know that your child has had a second seizure so that they can guide you regarding next steps in evaluation and possible treatment.

CHAPTER 7

Understanding Your Child's Tests
EEG, CT, and MRI

The physician's diagnosis of seizures or epilepsy is made only by reviewing the history of the episode or by seeing an episode. There is no "test for epilepsy."

Certain tests, such as the electroencephalogram (EEG) or long-term video-EEG monitoring can be helpful in determining the type of seizure and in assisting the physician to decide the type of medication to use. Scans of the brain, such as the CT scan or the MRI, can at times be useful in localizing an abnormality that may be causing the seizures. Since most children with epilepsy will have these tests on one or more occasions, it is helpful for you as a parent to understand the tests' utility and their limitations. First, the most common of such tests, the EEG.

The Electroencephalogram

We know that the firing of neurons in the brain is carefully modulated by the balance of excitation and inhibition of cells, and that groups of cells work together, interacting by exciting or inhibiting one another to coordinate everything that we think and do. The electroencephalogram (EEG) measures the electricity given off by the brain cells as they interact. The tiny amounts of electricity generated by the brain cells can be detected on the scalp, and if amplified many hundreds of times, this electricity can be transformed by the EEG machine and recorded (see Figures 7.1 and 7.2).

In most children without epilepsy, EEG recordings resemble wiggly

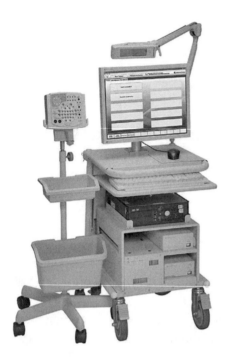

FIGURE 7.1. Modern EEG machine utilizing digitalized data collection. This form of collection allows for great flexibility in reading the records and ease in making the tracing available to multiple physicians.

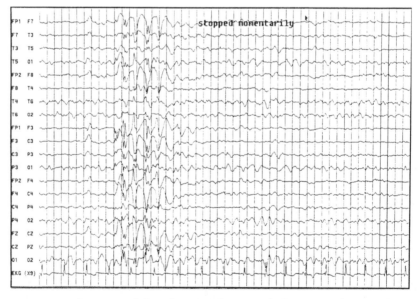

FIGURE 7.2. Printout of digital EEG. This record shows a spike-wave burst while a child was hyperventilating.

lines, the tiny waves varying slightly in height and frequency (see Figures 7.3 and 7.4). In most people with epilepsy, abnormalities can be seen on the EEG even in between seizures. These are little bursts of electrical activity, called *sharp waves* or *spikes*, that interrupt normal rhythm. These bursts are the result of the electrical discharge of a somewhat larger population of cells all firing simultaneously. They are not clinically detectable seizures, because the spikes and sharp waves do not represent enough cells firing simultaneously in a prolonged and unin-

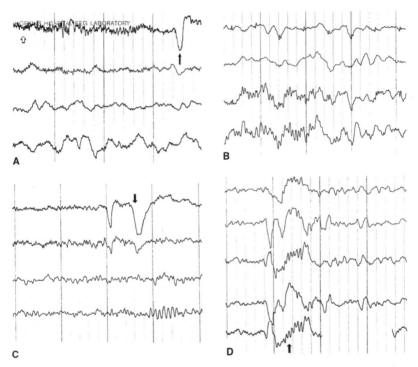

FIGURE 7.3. EEGs of normal infant and teenager. Record *A*, of an awake infant, shows blinking (*solid arrow*) and muscle artifact (*open arrow*), both in the first line, or channel. Much normal slowing is seen throughout the record. In *B*, the bottom two channels show the rhythmical fast activity, called spindles, of the infant when asleep; the two upper channels show a normal amount of slow activity that in many respects resembles the awake record. In the EEG of an awake teenager (*C*), when the eyes close (*arrow*), very rhythmical activity, known as the basic rhythm, appears in the bottom line; a sleep recording in the same teenager (*D*) shows a burst of activity (*arrow*) that is normal in sleep.

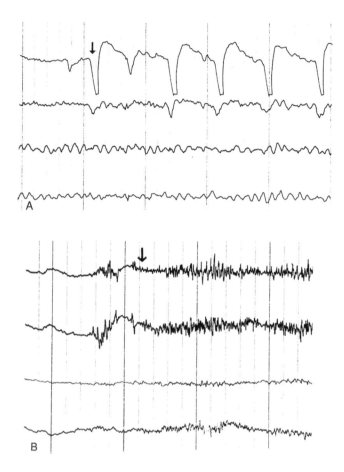

FIGURE 7.4. Normal EEG with eye movement and muscle artifacts. With the patient blinking (*A*), the top channel of the EEG record shows the eye movement (*arrow*). In *B*, the top two channels show muscle activity when the patient bites down or chews.

terrupted manner to alter the function or behavior of the person, but they indicate that the person's brain is more prone to having seizures. There is variability in how often this activity is present among different children and even in the same child at different times. Often even a 20-minute EEG will detect it, but this finding is not absolutely necessary to making a diagnosis of epilepsy and does not, alone, make the diagnosis. All EEG findings are interpreted in the context of each child's story.

When to Do an EEG

The first question to ask is, "Is this EEG really necessary?"

• Some EEGs are done to "rule out seizures." As discussed later in this chapter, EEGs do not rule out seizures, nor do they diagnose seizures.

• Sometimes EEGs are done every few months "to see how the child is doing," "to see if the medications are working," "to see if she is 'getting better.'" These are not good reasons for repeating the EEG if the child has not been having seizures.

• Some EEGs are repeated because the child's seizures are getting worse, breaking through the medication, or changing in character. These are good reasons to repeat the EEG.

• Sometimes the clinical picture of the child's seizures suggests that they come from one area of the brain. Documentation that there is a focal abnormality on the EEG is helpful to the physician in deciding what medication to use or whether to look for a focal abnormality using imaging of the brain.

• Certain patterns of abnormality of the EEG (spike and wave, focal or generalized slowing) may assist the physician in searching for a diagnosis or in choosing the best medication for the child's seizures. Looking for patterns is rarely a reason for frequent repetition of the EEG.

Performing an EEG

The EEG is best done with the child relaxed, sleepy, and still. The state of alertness may affect the EEG. Thus, crying, irritability, and restlessness may mask underlying abnormalities on the EEG and make it uninterpretable.

In the past we sedated many younger children for their EEGs, to avoid the movement and its artifacts and because we can often learn more if sleep is obtained. We now know that the effects of sedation can be mimicked if a few simple procedures are followed.

For the younger child

• Tell the child what is going to happen: that the technician will be putting some things in their hair, and that it will not hurt.

• Keep the child up late the night before the test and awaken them early. Do not let them sleep on the way to the test.

• Bring their favorite blanket, stuffed toy, or book so that they can hold it and feel comfortable.

• The EEG laboratory should be quiet and the technician calm, comfortable with children, and reassuring. If this is not the situation, you might consider asking if you can come back another time.

• The electrodes can often be pasted on while the child is in the parent's lap, and the EEG also may often be done with the child in your lap. This option may or may not be offered to you, depending on the practice of the laboratory you go to.

• We prefer that EEGs be done with the child both asleep and awake. This, too, is a matter of the specific doctor's preference or the specific laboratory's practice.

Older children usually need nothing more than an explanation of what is going to happen. The worst part of an EEG for them is getting the "gook" out of their hair after it is over.

Accompanying Your Child to the EEG

Usually, you may stay with your child to provide reassurance, but only if you are also quiet and still. Any movement and any touching or patting your child may cause electrical disturbances that show up on this sensitive machine and will confuse the EEG tracing. A child's muscle movements—crying, squirming, squeezing the eyes shut, or clenching the teeth—can cause the EEG machine to "go crazy" as it picks up the electricity from the muscles. Relaxation and quiet for both parent and child are crucial to a good recording.

Special EEG Procedures

Three special procedures that may be part of the routine EEG—sleep induction, hyperventilation, and photic stimulation—are called *activation procedures*, because they can activate patterns of abnormalities on the EEG. Such procedures should be routine with children.

Q. *"Why do they do the test both awake and asleep?"*
A. The EEG looks quite different depending on whether the patient is awake or asleep (Figure 7.5). Some abnormalities, spikes for example, may be apparent only in a drowsy or sleeping state because sleep changes the organization of brain waves and may allow hidden abnormalities to

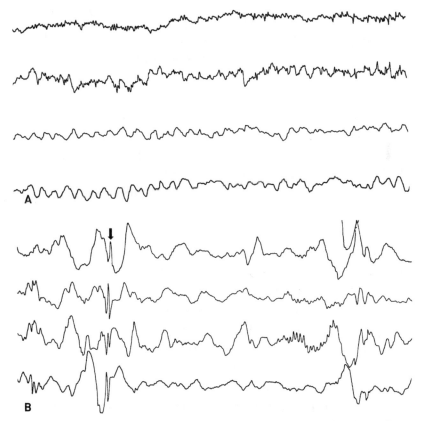

FIGURE 7.5. *A*, awake EEG of a 3-year-old. *B*, the same 3-year-old asleep, showing spike activity (*arrow*).

show up. Some children with epilepsy may have a normal EEG awake and a very abnormal EEG when asleep.

Q. *"What is hyperventilation, and why is it done?"*
A. The technician will ask your child to breathe deeply and rapidly, thus causing changes in the blood carbon dioxide and usually resulting in slowing on the EEG. Such changes as a consequence of hyperventilating are far more pronounced in younger children than in older ones. They can reveal abnormalities on the EEG. In children with absence seizures, over-breathing can even cause a clinical seizure and allow the EEG characteristics of this form of epilepsy to become overt.

Q. *"What is photic stimulation?"*
A. Flashing lights may also trigger seizures. You have heard about this when you have been warned about flashing lights on TV or movies. A special class of seizures is called *photic sensitive seizures*. Using a stroboscopic light, which flashes at frequencies from 1 per second to 60 per second, the EEG technician can observe whether the child is *photic sensitive*, that is, that the child's EEG responds to certain frequencies of flashes, with the EEG showing spikes every time the light flashes. Occasionally, *photic driving* can make the brain so active that a real seizure will occur, one similar to episodes that occur under nonlaboratory conditions in a few people. These people are said to have *photic sensitive epilepsy*.

Normal and Abnormal EEG Findings

Most of the lines and waveforms on any EEG are common and normal (see Figure 7.3). Some are the result of brain activity, and some are the result of electrical activity or movement outside the brain. When muscles twitch or contract, they produce electricity, and this electricity is picked up on the EEG. When people blink their eyes (called an *eye movement artifact*), this movement is also seen on the EEG. *Artifact* means that the electrical impulse is not coming from the brain, so it does not count. (Eye movement artifact is shown in Figure 7.4A.) *Muscle artifacts* can be seen when children clench their teeth, for instance (Figure 7.4B). When a child is awake, we look for an ongoing pattern (background activity) that is normal in frequency and amplitude for their age and state of wakefulness or sleep. We also look for something called a basic rhythm (frequency) that is seen over the back of the head while the child is quiet with eyes closed. This tells us whether the brain appears to be functioning normally. Even during the process of falling asleep, changes are produced in the rhythm of the EEG (Figure 7.3D) that look like bursts of abnormal electrical activity. None of these changes in rate or rhythm on the EEG is abnormal, so don't worry.

Three abnormalities on the EEG are important in the diagnosis and management of seizures: spikes, slowing, and evidence of seizures. Each of these may be either focal (occurring in a specific part of the brain) or generalized (occurring all over all at once). Each has a different meaning.

Remember, a clinical seizure is an electrical discharge or series of electrical discharges from the brain that causes a change in movement or behavior. If there is no change in behavior or movement, this is not a clinical seizure. Some abnormalities on the EEG without associated clinical changes may be called *electrographic-only seizures*. Electrographic-only seizures are relatively rare, and the management may be different than for clinical seizures and often specific to each individual patient.

The EEG may

- show electrical changes that indicate either an electrical abnormality in one area of the brain or electrical abnormalities in many areas of the brain;

- indicate to your child's physician that a specific area of the brain is involved;

- help the physician determine the type of seizure your child had; and/or

- indicate which medication is likely to be most effective for controlling that type of seizure.

Diagnosis of seizures or epilepsy depends on an accurate interpretation of the events that have occurred. The diagnosis of a seizure or of epilepsy is not made by the EEG alone. Furthermore, an EEG does not diagnose or rule out epilepsy. Some people with abnormal EEGs never have seizures. Some people with seizures have normal EEGs except when a seizure is occurring.

Spikes

Since a clinical seizure requires that a sufficient number of brain cells fire together to cause the alteration in movement or behavior, one would expect this firing to cause a change in the electrical activity recorded on the EEG. That is exactly what does happen. The normal EEG (Figures 7.3 and 7.4) represents the controlled and integrated firing of brain cells. When the cells fire simultaneously and uncontrolled, however, they produce an electrical abnormality in the EEG called a *spike* (Figure 7.6A).

Although seizures typically involve spikes on EEG, a single spike alone is not likely a seizure. If the electrical disturbance causing the spike spread to involve more cells or became repetitive at a fast-enough frequency to change behavior, however, a true clinical seizure would occur. Repeated spikes coming from a particular area represent the local response to a provocation there, an epileptic focus or scar. In a child (or adult) who has had a focal seizure, spikes may indicate the area of the brain where the seizure started (Figure 7.6A). Multifocal spikes (Figure 7.6B), by comparison, suggest that there are many abnormal areas of the brain.

Slowing

The rhythm of the normal EEG varies with the child's age and differs depending on whether the child is awake, drowsy, or asleep. There are well-established limits for these normal variations in rate and rhythm. When the frequency of the waveforms on a child's EEG are slower than we would expect for that particular age, we refer to this as *slowing*. Slowing may be either focal (Figure 7.6C) or generalized (Figure 7.6D).

There are many causes of abnormal slowing, and the degree, timing, and location of the slowing can tell us some things about the underlying dysfunction in the brain that is causing it and the severity or reversibility of the problem. A common cause of slowing is a postictal state, due to the needed inhibition of the firing of cells after a seizure. Postictal

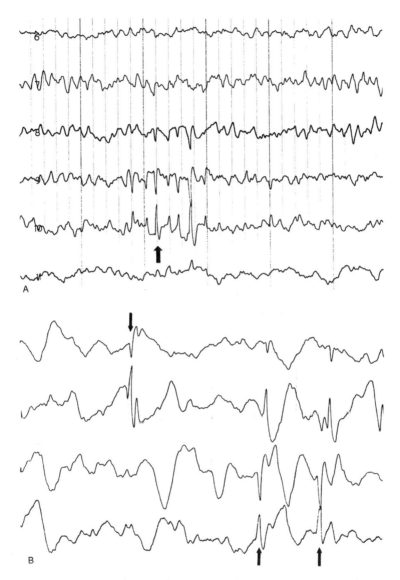

FIGURES 7.6A AND B. Abnormal EEGs. Each line, or channel, on the EEG represents a different area of the brain. In *A*, since the pointed spikes (*arrow*) shown in channels 9 and 10 do not appear in the other channels, the abnormality is focal in that specific area of the brain. In *B*, the multifocal spikes (*arrows*), appearing in several channels, show that they arise in several different areas of the brain and that there are multifocal abnormalities of the brain.

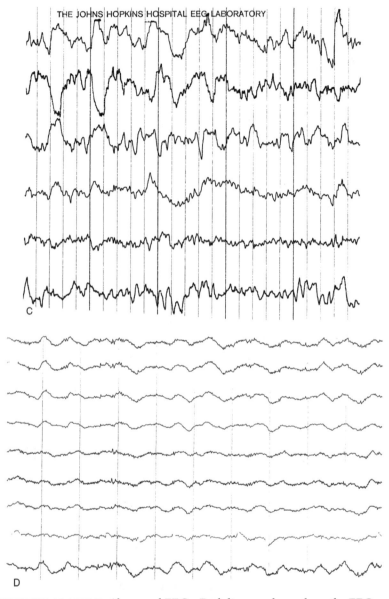

FIGURES 7.6C AND D. Abnormal EEGs. Each line, or channel, on the EEG represents a different area of the brain. In *C*, the top three channels (from left side of head) show high amplitude with slow waves, as compared to electrical activity from the right side of the head (*bottom three lines*). In *D*, all channels show low-voltage slow activity, as might be seen in a child in a coma.

slowing is best diagnosed by its temporal association with a seizure and its disappearance soon after the seizure, but it may last several hours. If slowing lasts for days after a seizure, further evaluation is necessary.

Focal slowing should always be of concern and requires careful evaluation because it may occur in association with a local disturbance of the brain, such as a concussion, a stroke, or a tumor. In a child who has had a seizure, persistent focal slowing on an EEG (unlike focal spikes, necessarily) may, therefore, require further imaging studies.

Slowing all over the brain—generalized slowing—signifies disturbed brain function caused by acute disturbances of whole brain function, as occurs in coma, chemical disturbances, lack of oxygen, infection, or severe head injury with loss of consciousness. Generalized slowing may also be seen in children with long-standing chronic brain dysfunction.

EEG Abnormalities Related to Certain Seizure Types

While the EEG does not diagnose seizures, certain abnormalities on the EEG are commonly associated with certain seizure types and can help your child's physician determine your child's treatment and the probable outcome. Thus, just as classification of seizures is useful, so is classification of EEGs.

Arjun is in the third grade and has been a very good student. But in the second half of the year, the teacher sends you a note that Arjun is not working up to his ability. He is not paying attention in class; he often daydreams. Sometimes, when he's asked a question, he claims that he didn't hear the question or that he has forgotten the answer. What's happening to Arjun? Is he bored and daydreaming? Is he not smart enough to understand the new work and, consequently, confused? Is he upset or depressed by events at home or school? Is he having staring spells (absence seizures)?

Absence Seizures

The EEG in a child with simple absence seizures often shows brief bursts of spike and wave abnormalities (Figure 7.7). In between these abnormalities, the background and basic rhythm is quite normal. Sometimes spontaneously, but usually with hyperventilation (over-breathing), the EEG demonstrates runs of spikes and waves, with a typical rate of three

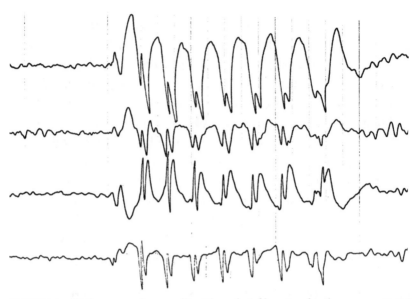

FIGURE 7.7. Spike-wave abnormality. These brief bursts of spike-wave activity, preceded and followed by normal activity, are often associated with absence seizures.

times a second. This type of electrical disturbance, if it lasts more than a few seconds, interferes with children's alertness or awareness. They will stare into space for a few seconds, then may say, "What? What did you say?" They return to their normal state just as quickly as they lost awareness. The EEG also abruptly returns to normal.

If Arjun has typical staring spells during hyperventilation and has a typical spike and wave pattern on his EEG, the physician will be able to tell his mother that these spells will probably be outgrown, that he is unlikely to develop other types of seizures, and that his seizures should respond easily to the right medication.

Atypical Absence Seizures

Atypical absence seizures are often difficult to differentiate from focal seizures with impaired awareness. The smaller the number of episodes per day, the earlier the age of onset, and, most particularly, what manifestations are associated with the seizure, such as lip smacking, picking at clothes, and confusion, may help identify the type of seizure. The EEG will often help distinguish between them, showing the classical three-per-second spike-wave of simple absence seizures and the somewhat slower spike-wave of atypical absence seizures.

Other Special Patterns

Hypsarrhythmia, a chaotic, high-voltage EEG pattern of spikes, po-ly-spikes, and slow waves seen in some children of six months to three years (Figure 7.8), is almost always associated with the severe seizure disorder infantile spasms (see Chapter 8). The Lennox-Gastaut pattern is also a pattern of slow spike-wave and poly-spikes as well as slow waves in multiple places on the EEG (Figure 7.9), a pattern seen in some children and young adults who have a mixed seizure disorder. The term is used to describe the EEG and also the seizure syndrome (see Chapter 8).

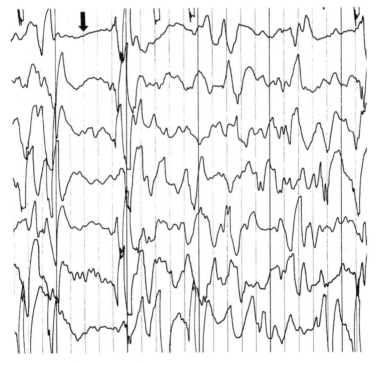

Figure 7.8. Hypsarrhythmic EEG, a chaotic, high-amplitude EEG with multifocal spikes, with a brief voltage suppression (*arrow*), usually seen in association with infantile spasms.

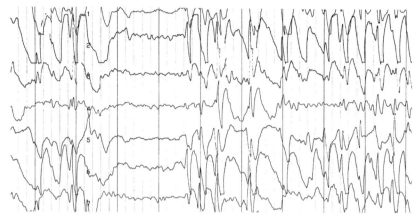

Figure 7.9. The Lennox-Gastaut pattern. Bursts of high-amplitude spikes and slow waves are less regular and well organized than the spike-wave activity of absence seizures.

Other types of epilepsy that can be diagnosed by a combination of the clinical pattern of the seizures and the EEG include childhood epilepsy with centro-temporal spikes (previously called benign childhood epilepsy with centro-temporal spikes or Rolandic epilepsy), which have central and midtemporal or parietal spikes, and juvenile myoclonic epilepsy (see Chapter 8).

Why Do an EEG?

"What will we learn from the EEG?" you ask. "You've said it doesn't diagnose epilepsy. You have stated that it does not rule out epilepsy. It sounds to me like it's useless, one of those tests you do because everyone does them and it looks like you're reading some message from the brain." Despite its limitations, the initial EEG is useful.

• Although it does not usually diagnose seizures, the EEG can be helpful in distinguishing between forms of epilepsy. The three-per-second spike-wave pattern of simple absence seizures, the chaotic pattern of hypsarrhythmia, or the Rolandic spikes of benign childhood epilepsy with centro-temporal spikes (to name a few patterns), when combined with the history and description of the episode, can identify the type of seizure. The physician can then suggest the best medications for that seizure type and can often predict the outcome of the seizures.

• A normal EEG, while not ruling out seizures, can be reassuring regarding the severity of the epilepsy if the child has recurrent spells.

• An abnormal EEG can suggest need for caution and increased awareness of recurrent spells.

• A focally abnormal EEG with either focal spikes or focal slowing can suggest the need for further evaluation with MRI scans.

• The EEG can serve as a baseline, so that if the seizures change in character, or get worse, there is something against which to compare future EEGs.

Why Repeat an EEG?

"If that's all they get out of the test, why would they want another one?" you might ask. Others might question, "Will the follow-up EEG really show that the epilepsy is getting better or worse?" The answer to both questions is that an EEG should be repeated only when it will provide useful information. It should not be repeated routinely, say, every three months, every six months, or even every year. If your child's seizures are controlled, you should not care if the EEG is normal or not—that is, until you want to consider stopping medication.

An EEG should be repeated only if

• seizures have been controlled for a significant period (usually 1–2 years) and the possibility of weaning medication is being considered; or

• seizures are continuing despite appropriate medication; or

• seizures are changing in pattern or frequency; or

• seizures that have been well controlled now recur; or

• the child's functioning/learning is changing. In that case it's really important to get a sleep EEG to see if there's a pattern of electrical status epilepticus of sleep (ESES).

In any of these circumstances, a change in the EEG could provide a clue to the reason for the change. A person who has had a few generalized tonic-clonic seizures, followed by successful control of seizures, might have only an initial EEG and no further EEGs unless the physician considers stopping medication, and then a second EEG may provide important information about the possibility of further seizures. A child who has frequent seizures or focal seizures might require many EEGs to determine where the seizures are coming from. A child with difficult-to-control seizures might also require many EEGs, or even continuous monitoring of the EEG for days, to capture the seizures as they occur and identify their origin in order to plan surgery. But continuous EEG monitoring, either with ambulatory (walking around) equipment or video monitoring, is a special test and should be used only in such special circumstances.

So, the answer to the question "Why repeat the EEG?" is that it depends. But if your child's physician wants a repeat, do not hesitate to ask why. They should be able and willing to tell you.

Intensive EEG Monitoring

For the evaluation of most individuals with epilepsy, no special EEG tests are required. For most such children, the neurological evaluation, one EEG, and in some cases an MRI scan will provide sufficient evaluation. Nonetheless, in three situations special EEG tests are indicated:

• If the episodes do not seem to fit any particular seizure type, your child's physician may be concerned that these are not true epileptic seizures caused by abnormal electrical activity in the brain, but rather are nonepileptic events or psychogenic nonepileptic seizures (PNES), previously referred to as pseudoseizures. Special EEG monitoring may help to separate epileptic seizures from PNES or other neurological and nonneurological episodes that mimic seizures.

• Special EEG monitoring is always required when surgery is even considered as a possible treatment for epilepsy. The testing may indicate that the seizures are coming from several different areas of the brain, thus making some types of surgery less likely to be effective. Alternatively, intensive monitoring may indicate sufficient evidence of a focal source for the seizures, and it may be worth initiating a series of additional tests that would help in making intelligent decisions about surgery (see Chapter 14).

• Some children with uncontrolled seizures may benefit from intensive monitoring that might identify the type of seizure and indicate the need for alternative medications.

Ambulatory EEG Monitoring

Ambulatory EEG monitoring uses portable EEG equipment to permit long-term constant monitoring of the EEG while a child is doing normal things—sleeping or out of bed, playing, at home, in school, or on the hospital ward. The advantage of ambulatory EEG monitoring is that it is relatively inexpensive, since it requires neither being in the hospital nor a lot of the supervisory personnel. Thus, it can be performed even when the seizures are of relatively low frequency. The disadvantages are that the physician may not be able to see the clinical episodes on video and cannot localize their onset. Ambulatory EEG monitoring is useful when:

• the physician needs to determine if the episodes the child is having are truly seizures. If the EEG does not show the electrical activity usually seen with a seizure, at the time of the episode, that can be evidence of some other reason for the episode. The converse may also be true, and episodes thought not to be seizures may indeed have the electrical signature of a seizure.

• there is a need to count the number of seizures the child is having. It is sometimes necessary to check the seizure frequency to correctly adjust treatment protocols.

Ambulatory EEG monitoring is not needed for every patient. It is rarely needed to diagnose or confirm epilepsy, and it is often overused. Various types of portable equipment can be used for this ambulatory monitoring. All require that the EEG electrodes be glued to the scalp and connected by wires to the recording device; electrodes becoming unglued is the major problem with this form of monitoring. The wires are run to a small device worn on the patient, which records the electrical activity. Some monitoring systems include a home computer, which can be plugged into the monitor and will store even more information and even recognize seizures.

The biggest problem with this monitoring (other than the electrodes coming loose) is that the parents must indicate when the events occur, by pushing a button, and must describe each event on a log sheet. If the parents do not push the button, then even if there is an electrical change on the EEG, the reader of the data record does not know if the child had a clinical event or not. If the parent pushes the button and records what is occurring with the child, then we can see if there was an electrical correlate. Some of the newer computerized recording devices have spike detectors, which detect the electrical activity often associated with seizures. While this permits detection of events that the parents do not see (like brief seizures occurring during the night), it also detects the many artifacts that accompany movement and muscle activity, and this density of information makes the recording more difficult and cumbersome to read.

While ambulatory EEG monitoring permits recognition of major brain abnormalities, such as generalized spike and wave seizures, it is not precise enough for presurgical evaluations. There are additional drawbacks and limitations to ambulatory monitoring, and because the child is monitored at home and it is not uncommon for one or more of the electrodes to become loose without anyone knowing, the monitoring may yield less than accurate reports. It may be impossible to interpret any episodes that occur if some of the electrodes are not working. When used appropriately, however, ambulatory EEG monitors can be exceedingly helpful in selected cases.

Video-EEG Monitoring

The optimal approach to analysis of seizures is to both see and record their onset and their spread. Such an approach is mandatory in situations in which surgery is being considered. When determining if surgery is even an option, it is critical to know the exact area of the brain involved in the origin of the seizures. Video-EEG monitoring allows recording of the EEG from multiple areas of the brain and simultaneous video recording of the seizures. Ideally this is performed in an epilepsy monitoring unit (EMU), a specialized inpatient hospital unit where staff are trained to effectively operate video and EEG monitoring equipment as well as to manage medications and induction techniques so that seizures can be captured during the monitoring period (Figure 7.10). Additionally, the interactions of trained staff with the child during a seizure can provide additional useful clinical information about the seizures.

Video-EEG monitoring can also be useful when there is a question about what the spells really are. The ability to see a spell that is said to be a seizure and to interact with the patient and record the EEG at the same time is the definitive way to differentiate seizures from PNES.

Two examples will illustrate what we're talking about.

• *Kim was a 15-year-old with a severe behavioral disorder and seizures. Despite several years of intensive outpatient psychotherapy, she was once again thrown out of school. Her family was exasperated. It was clear to both her neurologist and her psychiatrist that she used her*

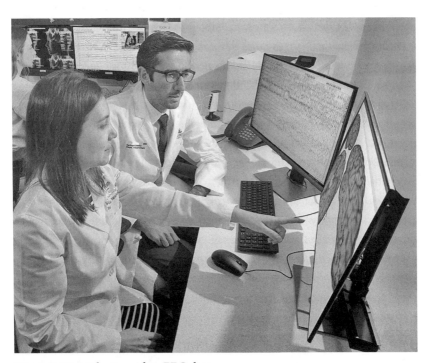

Figure 7.10 Analyzing video-EEG data.

seizures to manipulate her environment. She was taken off medication, and these peculiar episodes, which did not sound like seizures, did not increase in frequency. The family was taught to ignore them, and Kim seemed able to control them. But their persistence and her abnormal EEG remained of concern to her psychiatrist. The only resolution to this problem was to send her to a residential institution where she could be taught better behavioral control. Since the psychiatrist at the institution was uncomfortable dealing with a child with seizures, we brought her into the monitoring unit to see whether all her spells were PNES. Much to our surprise, while most of her episodes were, indeed, PNES, at night she had genuine tonic-clonic seizures. Placing her back on medication eliminated these true seizures and allowed the psychiatrist at the institution to concentrate on her behavioral problems. It's important to remember that a significant number of people with PNES also have actual seizures with EEG abnormalities.

• Simon's seizures began when he was 2 years old. They would start in his left foot and spread up the left side. At times, he would have a weakness in the left leg that was thought to be postictal paralysis, but at other times, the leg was quite normal. Despite intensive attempts with medication, seizures continued to occur several times each day. The EEG showed a focus near the motor strip on the right, and we faced the choice of operating to remove the focus (with the probability of causing paralysis at least of the leg) or of allowing him to continue to have seizures. We decided to wait. After several years, video-EEG monitoring allowed us to see the start of several seizures. They actually began anteriorly in the frontal lobe and then spread into the motor strip. They began in an area that could possibly be removed without damaging his motor ability. Simon was, therefore, put on the list for evaluation, with the grid electrodes placed on the surface of his brain (see Chapter 14), and eventually had successful surgery—without experiencing paralysis.

Intensive monitoring allows us to make decisions that would be difficult to make without actually seeing the episode and understanding whether EEG changes are associated with it and where those changes come from. It gives us the opportunity to separate true seizures definitively from PNES and, importantly, to identify children as prospects for surgery. Not everyone needs video-EEG monitoring. Only if an important question must be resolved is the expense and inconvenience for the family warranted. If there is a question regarding surgery, this monitoring should be done at a center capable of doing the surgery. It is difficult, or impossible, for surgical decisions to be made based on tests conducted and interpreted by others.

Many epilepsy centers are capable of intensive video-EEG monitoring. Video-EEG monitoring is usually carried out in special hospital settings with the patient in bed or sitting in a chair where the video camera and EEG machine can constantly monitor their activities. The EEG and the video are recorded simultaneously in one of several ways that will permit simultaneous analysis of the behavior and the electrical activity. Often these intensive monitoring centers will withdraw medication to precipitate seizures, which can then be recorded. Staff are specially trained to keep children safe during these seizures. Information about the availability and nature of the services offered by centers is available at the National Association of Epilepsy Centers' website (https://www .naec-epilepsy.org/).

The principal drawback to this monitoring is its expense. It requires the use of hospital space and the time of nurses or technicians who will monitor the patient and the equipment 24 hours a day. Also, analysis of the records (Figure 7.10) is expensive and time consuming. Because seizures must be of sufficient frequency to make their recording feasible, intensive video-EEG monitoring may require many days in the EMU at enormous cost. Video-EEG monitoring is sometimes used on an outpatient basis in an EEG lab for 8 to 12 hours. When spells are sufficiently frequent, this abbreviated monitoring may be adequate and is much less expensive.

Yet, when seizures are sufficiently frequent and disabling to the individual, or when the localization of the onset of seizures is sufficiently important to future decision making about medication or surgery, then intensive monitoring, expensive as it is, is cost effective. The goals of hospital admission and monitoring must, of course, be carefully defined in advance to make the most efficient use of this complex system.

CT and MRI Scanning

"Dave, I'm so glad you called. I didn't know where to reach you. Joel had a seizure. I thought he was going to die. We had had a good day; he had a friend over and they played nicely. I'd read him a story and put him to sleep in our bed, since you were out of town. I don't know what made me go back and check; maybe I heard a noise. Joel was choking. He was stiff and jerking. I didn't know what to do. I put him on his side and called 911. By the time they arrived, the jerking and choking were over, and Joel seemed to be sleeping. The EMTs put in an IV and took us to the emergency room. The nurses there took some blood and sent him down for a CT scan, and by the time that was done, a doctor had arrived, and Joel was awake. The doctor said that Joel had had a seizure but that his blood work looked okay. He said we didn't need to do a spinal tap because he didn't have a fever, and the CT scan was okay, but he wanted an MRI done on Friday. He said it was to rule out a tumor or something causing the seizure. Can you be back home by Friday? I'm scared."

When a child has had a seizure or multiple seizures, the first question parents and physicians ask is, "Why did the seizure occur?" Although most seizures in children are *idiopathic* or *genetic* (having no known cause or genetically determined), and although most that are symptomatic (due to a structural or chemical disturbance in the brain) are secondary to something that happened long ago, there is an almost irresistible urge among physicians and families to "take a look," to see if "we can find out why this occurred." Neurologists and neurosurgeons who see adults who have just begun to have frequent seizures appropriately consider brain tumors or vascular (blood vessel) problems as a possible cause of these seizures. The causes of seizures in children are different. Tumors and vascular problems are rarely the cause of new onset seizures in children.

Modern radiology has made it possible to "take a look" inside the brain relatively easily, at modest expense and without significant harm to the patient. Nonetheless, it is not necessary to obtain an image of the brain of every child who has had a first seizure. There are good reasons for a physician to request a scan if:

• there are repeated focal seizures, or

• there is focal slowing on the EEG, or

• you or your child's physician are concerned that your child is getting worse.

In such circumstances, the main reason to obtain an image of your child's brain is to determine if there is a progressive process (as is the case with tumors) that may require intervention. Alternatively, in the case of the child getting worse despite treatment, it may help to make a specific diagnosis with specific treatment.

Yet, it is important to remember:

• Most scans are normal in children with epilepsy.

• Most abnormalities found will not explain the epilepsy.

• Most abnormalities found will not lead to a different approach to treatment.

Just because something abnormal is seen on an image, it does not mean that this abnormality has caused the seizure or seizures or that it will cause seizures in the future. Only if the abnormality on the scan appears in the proper location of the brain to have caused the seizures can we presume cause and effect. The most common changes are nonspecific findings or evidence of an injury that occurred in the remote past.

CT Scanning

CT or CAT scanning (computerized tomography or computerized axial tomography), a procedure introduced in the early 1970s, at the time revolutionized the ability to "see" the brain. Low-dose X-rays are detected and interpreted by a computer, which then generates a picture just as if we had cut a slice of the brain. CT scans are relatively good at detecting large injuries, aggressive tumors, and blood but are not as good at detecting more subtle abnormalities, and they expose your child to radiation. This is the reason we frequently don't recommend this type of study, even though it can be done quickly. The principal reason for doing a CT scan is to see whether the seizure had a cause that needs to be treated surgically and immediately. Otherwise, magnetic resonance imaging (MRI) gives far more information.

Why a CT Scan?

The evaluation of a seizure in the emergency room seems always to include blood work and a CT scan. Why? Perhaps to rule out any head trauma as a cause, although a history could usually rule that out. To rule out a tumor, a stroke, or a clot? Again, in a previously healthy child, a seizure is rarely the first sign of such an event, particularly if they have returned to their baseline normal exam after the seizure.

- In a child who has not had head trauma, an emergency CT is virtually never useful but is quickly obtainable and relatively inexpensive.

- An MRI is able to show small and subtle abnormalities that are not seen on the CT scan.

An MRI is always preferable to a CT scan if any scan is needed. The MRI is usually done after the CT, "to be sure," and the CT is then superfluous, except in the case of suspected head trauma. It is therefore a general recommendation that if a child has otherwise returned to their normal baseline after a seizure and the history does not suggest an acute process that needs to be immediately tended to, the providers should avoid the extra radiation of a CT scan and wait to obtain an MRI.

MRI Scanning

While CT scanning originally revolutionized our ability to see the brain, magnetic resonance imaging (MRI) has increased our ability to see the brain even more clearly. Unlike CT scanning, MRI does not employ X-rays but uses a huge magnet to create an image, which is then analyzed by computer as the CT is. It produces pictures of far greater detail, and with the exception of certain emergency management situations, MRI has largely replaced CT scans in the evaluation and management of epilepsy.

The principal disadvantages of MRI are that, with current equipment, an MRI scan usually takes a much longer time, during which the child must lie perfectly still in the tunnel-like machine and thus may require sedation. The test is more expensive than computerized tomography. Nonetheless, when detail of the brain is important, or when subtle changes must be seen, the MRI is indicated. It produces far better pictures of the brain and of most abnormalities than the CT scan does. If it is important to look for an acute abnormality in a sick child who has just had a seizure, the CT scan may be faster and cheaper. Such screening is rarely needed, however, and at many medical centers, rapid MRI scan protocols can replace CTs. If the person is having repeated focal seizures, and an abnormality has not been obvious on CT scanning, MRI scanning may show subtle abnormalities causing the seizures. As mentioned above, this type of study may require sedation for the younger child, and the process of sedating a child comes with its own risks. At most pediatric specialty hospitals, however, this type of sedation is routinely performed and safe, but it is always important to discuss the specific risks that may be unique to your child.

If your child's physician wants them to have an EEG or an MRI scan, you should feel free to ask why they want the test and what they hope to learn from it. These questions are even more appropriate if they want to repeat the test. Depending on the child's age, the need for sedation during an MRI may be the biggest risk of doing the test. It is always appropriate to discuss with your child's providers whether there is the possibility of attempting the study without sedation and using behavioral relaxation techniques.

Other scanning techniques, such as magnetic resonance spectroscopy (MRS), functional MRI (fMRI), single photon emission spectroscopy (SPECT), magnetoencephalography (MEG), and proton emission tomography (PET), are specialized methods that are not part of the initial work-up for a seizure. They are used when seizures are persistent and when the epilepsy team is searching for a single source of origin for the seizures, a source that might be amenable to surgery. These techniques are discussed in Chapter 14 about the surgical evaluation of seizures.

CHAPTER 8

The Epilepsies of Childhood, Part I

Special Patterns

Epilepsy and Its Special Forms

Epilepsy is defined as two or more seizures that are not due to an acute disturbance of the brain *or* one unprovoked seizure along with evidence on EEG or otherwise that the child has a predisposition to repeated seizures. Because there are many different types of seizures, epilepsy can take many different forms. There is not, thus, one epilepsy but many. Therefore, if we were to speak properly, we would not speak about "epilepsy" but about "the epilepsies or epilepsy syndromes."

Epilepsy Syndromes

In addition to the many types of seizures discussed in Chapter 2, various patterns of recurrent seizures are sufficiently distinctive in their course and outcome and in their response to specific medications to warrant distinct names and separate discussions. In general, these syndromes range from benign syndromes with good overall outcomes to those that may be more severe and associated with developmental disorders. Recognizing and understanding the epilepsy syndromes, in general, provides some broad guidance regarding treatment and prognosis. It can help families understand the bigger picture of how their child's epilepsy may evolve and be treated. It can also connect them to other parents and resources. Nonetheless, it is important to recognize that no matter what your child's specific diagnosis is, each child is a unique individual who will fall somewhere within a range of symptoms and severity even within a specific syndrome. The list of syndromes discussed below is not inclusive of all epilepsy syndromes. These particular syndromes are discussed because they are the most commonly diagnosed epilepsy syndromes in childhood or because their distinctive features or severity makes them more likely to be recognized.

Childhood Epilepsy with Centrotemporal Spikes

Previously known as benign childhood epilepsy with centrotemporal spikes (BCECTS) or benign rolandic epilepsy, childhood epilepsy with centrotemporal spikes (CECTS) is a special form of epilepsy in children, typically starting after 3 years of age (average age of onset 7–9 years), and the most prevalent epilepsy syndrome of childhood. It accounts for about 10–20 percent of childhood epilepsy. It has typical clinical manifestations and a typical EEG. It is usually "benign" in that the seizures are outgrown at adolescence whether or not it is treated and in that the children are usually developing typically before, during, and after the years during which they may have seizures. In many or most cases, the seizures are infrequent and do not necessarily need treatment with medication. If a child's seizures are more frequent or troublesome, treatment can be highly effective and may be tapered and discontinued after puberty.

Seizures in this form of epilepsy often start with a sensation at the corner of the mouth, which is followed by jerking of that corner. The jerking may stay on one side of the face or spread to the other and can cause a twisting of the affected side of the face. There may also be drooling and slurred speech along with the jerking, or after the movement has stopped. The seizure may, on occasion, spread throughout that side of the body, affecting the arms and legs, or spread throughout both sides and become a generalized tonic-clonic seizure. These seizures occur more commonly at night and during certain stages of sleep but can occur during the daytime as well.

The diagnosis of CECTS is confirmed by an EEG pattern of repetitive spike activity firing from the midtemporal, central, or parietal areas of the brain near the rolandic (motor) strip—hence the original name of benign rolandic epilepsy. Bilateral spike activity on the EEG is not uncommon, and interictal activity is more common on the EEG during certain stages of sleep.

There is a genetic predisposition to this form of epilepsy, and specific genes have been associated with the syndrome in some families, but genetic testing is generally not undertaken unless there is a particular family history or an atypical course. Imaging of the brain is generally not necessary, although an MRI may be ordered by your child's provider if there are specific concerns on exam or the EEG or seizure pattern is not classic, in order to rule out a symptomatic epilepsy (epilepsy caused by another pathologic process) that mimics CECTS. Some children with CECTS may develop difficulty with language and reading. Although these are rare cases, your child's physician should screen for difficulty and may recommend more formal neuropsychological testing if there are concerns.

Benign Occipital Epilepsies of Childhood

Panayiotopoulos syndrome, previously known as early onset benign occipital epilepsy of childhood (BOEC), is another common epilepsy syndrome affecting approximately 6 percent of children with epilepsy under age 15 years. Most children with Panayiotopoulos syndrome develop seizures between 3 and 6 years of age. This syndrome is characterized by seizures that present as abnormal activity of the autonomic nervous system, which has unconscious control over most organ systems. Typical seizures occur at night out of sleep and involve nausea, retching, or vomiting and behavioral changes. Other features that occur instead of, or along with, these emetic symptoms can include pallor or flushing of the skin, changes in pupils, deviation of the eyes to one side, changes in breathing, increased heart rate, headache, drooling or coughing, as well as other autonomic symptoms.

Seizures can be exceptionally long, lasting more than 30 minutes, and can progress to altered awareness and one-sided (hemi) tonic-clonic or generalized tonic-clonic seizures. Although these can be frightening to children and parents, the seizures are typically very rare, with many children having only a single seizure and most having them so infrequently that daily medications are usually not necessary. A rescue medication to be given during and used to stop prolonged seizures may be prescribed. This type of epilepsy usually occurs in otherwise typically developing children, and most children outgrow the seizures within two years of onset, with continued typical development during and after the period of seizures. Interestingly, the EEG in these children is similar to that of children with CECTS, although there may be more prominent discharges in the posterior or occipital part of the brain, as the name indicates.

Childhood occipital epilepsy (Gastaut-type) is much rarer and has a wide range of onset, with the peak at 8.5 years. Simple visual hallucinations or transient blindness and progression to gaze deviation (looking to one side) are the most characteristic seizure symptoms, and often children report headaches afterward. Seizures are much more frequent than in BOEC and can occur multiple times a day without medication, but they are short, lasting seconds to minutes. Not all children will outgrow them, but more than half of children will.

Childhood and Juvenile Absence Epilepsies

Childhood absence epilepsy (CAE) is one of the most common epilepsy diagnoses in childhood, making up 10–17 percent of epilepsy diagnoses in children under age 16. Because of the frequency as well as the number of seizures that children with this diagnosis have, it is one of the most recognizable epilepsies. It is most often diagnosed in typically developing school-aged children. Seizures start between 4 and 10 years, most commonly between 5 and 7 years. The predominant seizure type is a short (5–20 seconds long) absence seizure, occurring dozens to hundreds of times a day. As described in Chapter 7 these are characterized by brief activity arrest or staring and sometimes automatic behaviors, such as blinking, licking lips, or fumbling with hands. Some children will also have generalized tonic-clonic seizures or myoclonic seizures (jerks), but the predominant seizure type is absence.

The first-line treatment for CAE is ethosuximide, which is generally well tolerated, but valproic acid, lamotrigine, and possibly zonisamide have similar effectiveness and may be more helpful if children have generalized tonic-clonic seizures as well. Most children with CAE will respond to medications and eventually outgrow their seizures. Although in general, children with CAE have normal cognition, studies have shown higher rates of attention deficit hyperactivity disorder (ADHD) and behavioral or psychological problems compared to children without epilepsy, and screening for these comorbidities is important.

Juvenile absence epilepsy (JAE) begins later in childhood, around the time of puberty onset. Compared to CAE, children with JAE are more likely to have generalized tonic-clonic seizures and myoclonic seizures. Absences may not be as frequent or prominent. Seizures are less likely to be outgrown, but a third of children will eventually outgrow them.

Juvenile Myoclonic Epilepsy

Juvenile myoclonic epilepsy (JME) starts in late childhood or adolescence, often about the time of puberty. It accounts for 5–10 percent of all epilepsy. Its hallmark is mild myoclonic jerks, most common as the person is going to sleep or waking in the morning. An adolescent will describe jerking of the arms or legs, a feeling of being jumpy. If a person has early morning jerkiness, informing their doctor about the jerks may make it easier to diagnosis this particular form of epilepsy.

Some patients have told us that they set their alarm clocks to wake up early and then stay in bed for a half-hour to an hour, until the jumpiness wears off. They say that if they get up more quickly, the jerking gets much worse. Occasionally, the jerking increases and becomes sufficiently severe that the person experiences a clonic or a tonic-clonic seizure. In addition, people with juvenile myoclonic epilepsy may experience absence seizures, and there can sometimes be overlap between JME and JAE.

The EEG between seizures, in this form of epilepsy, often shows a fast, multiple- or double-spike (poly-spike) pattern followed by slow waves, with fast rapid spikes occurring during the jerks. When the diagnosis is suspected, the best way of confirming it is a sleep EEG, continued for 10 or 15 minutes after the person awakens. It is during this time that the jerks and the characteristic EEG pattern are most likely to be seen, but the diagnosis can also be made based on a routine EEG and a consistent history.

Diagnosis is important because, although this form of epilepsy responds poorly to many medications, it is usually easily controlled with valproic acid. In young women, for whom valproic acid poses a significant risk of teratogenicity and other side effects including polycystic ovary syndrome, lamotrigine and levetiracetam are often effective. This type of epilepsy is usually *not* outgrown and may require lifelong medication. A history of epilepsy may occur in as many as 40 percent of siblings of those with JME. The underlying cause is believed to be genetic. Although multiple different genes have been implicated in some families, however, the genetic basis is still not completely understood for most.

Infantile Spasms (West Syndrome)

West syndrome is a special form of epilepsy that starts in infancy, is readily recognized clinically, but initially may be mistaken for colic or reflux or perhaps a movement disorder. The characteristic seizures of this syndrome are infantile spasms. They account for about 2 percent of childhood epilepsy. During a typical infantile spasm, the child will suddenly flex their head or their body at the waist. The arms come up in a startle-like reaction, the knees are drawn up, and the child may let out a short cry. This spasm lasts just a second or two, then the child relaxes, but the spasm quickly recurs in the same form. These spasms continue in a series of five to fifty or more before the series stops. The child may have many series per day.

Since the child's mother often thinks that the cry and the flexion represent cramps or pain, her description may sound to the physician as if the child has colic, but *colic does not occur in a series of episodes.* Less frequently, as opposed to the flexor spams described above, the spasms may be extensor, with the head thrown back and the body briefly stiffening while the legs are extended; or the spasm may be unilateral, with one arm coming up, the head turned to that side, and the leg on the same side extended. These brief atypical spells also occur in series. Often the child appears distressed by what is happening.

Infantile spasms are the only type of seizures in which seizures occur in a defined series. The series, or cluster, of infantile spasms is most likely to occur when the child is drowsy, either waking from a nap or going to sleep. A parent might notice them particularly when the child has been placed in a highchair for a meal. Infantile spasms rarely start before 2 months of age or after a year and most commonly begin between 4 and 8 months. Spells that occur in a series, or cluster, in this age group are usually infantile spasms or one of its variants.

Even untreated, this form of epilepsy gradually disappears during the second to the fourth year of life. Nonetheless, the child often becomes developmentally delayed and may develop other seizure types. Shortly after the spasms begin, these children seem to stop making developmental progress and often lose skills they had previously acquired. A child who had started to sit may stop sitting, may even lose the ability to roll over, may stop babbling, and may function like a much younger child. Because of this deterioration, children with infantile spasms are often thought to have an underlying degeneration of the brain. Only 10 to 20 percent of children with infantile spasms will have normal neurodevelopmental function; the vast majority will have moderate to severe neurodevelopmental disability.

This is the *only* seizure type for which one can predict such a poor outlook (prognosis). The poor prognosis is in part a consequence of the underlying brain pathology that causes the spasms, but it may also in some way be a result of the effects of chaotic electrical activity in the brain. Some people think that the earlier the treatment of these seizures is initiated, the better the outlook. But even infants whose spasms are brought under control with treatment often develop another special form of epilepsy called Lennox-Gastaut syndrome.

Infantile spasms may occur in the young child who has developmental problems of the brain due to certain genetic changes or with brain damage caused by birth injury, meningitis, or head trauma. Abnormalities of sugar or amino acid metabolism, among other things, may also be responsible. All of these are designated "symptomatic" infantile spasms since they are caused by the underlying process. Many of these patients will have seizures or other neurological symptoms prior to the onset of the spasms. Despite discovering the cause for infantile spasms with modern-day testing, there remains a second and smaller group of infantile spasms that are called *cryptogenic*, meaning hidden, even when extensive testing has been done, since their cause is unknown. Children with cryptogenic infantile spasms appear perfectly normal in development before the seizures begin and may be more likely to respond to treatment and have typical or relatively typical developmental outcomes.

Infantile spasms are virtually always accompanied by an abnormality of the EEG known as *hypsarrhythmia*, a wildly chaotic high-voltage pattern with multiple spikes and slow waves. A useful analogy is to think of this EEG pattern as imposing severe "static" on the brain waves so that the brain functions poorly and the child's functioning deteriorates.

A physician evaluating a child with infantile spasms should search for treatable metabolic causes of the spasms and infectious processes. An EEG and an MRI scan should also be requested. Unless a specific treatable condition is found, and one rarely is, standard treatment for the spasms should begin promptly.

Although ACTH (adrenocorticotropic hormone), a form of steroid given twice a day by intramuscular injection, has been the standard treatment, some physicians use the oral steroid prednisolone. Overall, studies comparing the two treatments do not demonstrate that one is superior to the other, and because of the extremely excessive cost of ACTH, prednisolone is more readily accessible. In certain cases, such as infantile spasms due to tuberous sclerosis (discussed in the next chapter), vigabatrin may be the treatment of choice. The ketogenic diet (see Chapter 12) may also be considered for treatment if the diagnosis is made within a week or two of the onset of spasms. In children who fail to respond to standard therapies, other medications such as topiramate, valproic acid, or benzodiazepines may be tried. Each treatment has side effects, but there are also substantial risks in not treating this form of epilepsy.

Lennox-Gastaut Syndrome

Lennox-Gastaut syndrome, named after the two epileptologists who described its various components, is characterized by two or more types of seizures, a particular EEG pattern of diffuse spike or poly-spike and slow waves, and by global developmental delay or intellectual disability. The syndrome usually begins between the ages of 2 and 6, often in children who previously had infantile spasms. It accounts for 2–4 percent of childhood epilepsy. As with infantile spasms, there is no known single cause, but the syndrome commonly arises in children with developmental problems of the brain due to genetic factors or acquired brain damage. It is important to search for a degenerative and potentially treatable process that may be causing the seizures. Cryptogenic cases, ones for which no cause is found, may have a somewhat better prognosis than cases in children whose seizures are symptomatic of a known disease process.

Children with the Lennox-Gastaut syndrome commonly experience multiple seizure types. In the most disabling seizures, children suddenly fall to the ground, either forward or, less often, backward, frequently injuring themselves. Many of these children are forced to wear helmets with face masks to protect their teeth and faces from trauma. In addition, tonic seizures and atypical absence seizures are common, with occasional tonic-clonic seizures as well.

Children with these multiple, difficult-to-control seizures are often given several simultaneous medications with resulting medication side effects as well. The handicapping nature of the seizures, plus the drug toxicity and the continuous electrical abnormalities on the EEG, often reinforce the intrinsic brain dysfunction and result in significant incapacitation of the child. It's always important to try to weigh the risks and the benefits of adding antiseizure medications. It's critical to assess whether an added medication made the seizures better or only added side effects.

Despite this dismal outlook, some children respond well to medications. Some end up with little or no disability. Some have their seizures controlled with newer medications or with the ketogenic diet. Parents often despair when they hear the term Lennox-Gastaut applied to their child's EEG or seizures, but as with most diagnoses in medicine, there is a range of outcomes. As with infantile spasms, Lennox-Gastaut syndrome is a most frustrating and devastating condition. This group of children make up a large proportion of the intractable seizure population. Research is needed to understand their condition and to develop better forms of therapy. The frustration involved in their management and the complexity of treatment lead us to suggest that these children be evaluated and managed under the consultation of sophisticated epilepsy centers with access to newer medications.

Landau-Kleffner Syndrome and Other Language Impairments

Back in the "old days" we thought we understood a condition called Landau-Kleffner syndrome, a rare malady in which children would usually develop mild seizures and then gradually lose language, first the understanding of language and later speech production. These children always had EEG abnormalities that were often most marked in the speech area over the left temporal regions. It was widely believed that this syndrome was due to *epileptic aphasia* (lack of speech, due to epilepsy). At times, the EEG during sleep showed electrical status epilepticus (electrical status epilepticus of sleep, or ESES), defined as having seizure activity during the majority of the sleep recording. The natural history of this condition was grim. Many of these children did not recover speech for years. Many of them became mildly to moderately intellectually disabled.

Now we recognize a spectrum of severity, with some children having ESES on EEG but generally neurotypical development. Others have a subacute progressive loss of language associated with EEG abnormalities, as described for Landau-Kleffner syndrome. Still others with ESES on EEG and clinical seizures have mild to severe impairments and regression in not just language but in other areas of development as well. When there are cognitive changes, the term *continuous spike and wave in sleep* (CSWS) is often used. Often at diagnosis, it is not easy to predict what the course of an individual child will be, and regular follow-up and neurocognitive assessments are essential to track development and potentially response to treatment.

Various antiseizure medications, including valproic acid, benzodiazepines, and levetiracetam, steroids, and surgery have been reported to be successful in normalizing the sleep EEG and bringing speech and cognitive performance back to near the levels of typical peers in some, but not in all, children with this condition. Multiple underlying causes include various genetic changes and brain injuries, and it is likely that different causes may have different prognoses and responses to treatment. There are no standard treatment regimens at this point and no standard way to predict who will respond; formal studies are needed on both underlying causes and rational approaches to treatment.

There continues to be confusion related to this topic and that of other language and cognitive developmental disorders. If children who previously had language lose language due to abnormal electrical activity in the speech area, they are said to have Landau-Kleffner syndrome. If the same process were to occur *before* speech was present, presumably speech would not develop and so could not be lost. Would this be Landau-Kleffner-like? Lack of speech can also be due to developmental problems of the brain. These problems may be associated with abnormal EEGs and even with seizures but are not necessarily caused by them. Rather, the changes on EEG, seizures, and speech problems may all be the result of the same underlying changes in brain development.

Developmental delays, impairment of speech production, and varying degrees of intellectual impairment are often associated with autism spectrum disorders (ASDs). Thus ASD, some forms of intellectual disability (ID), and Landau-Kleffner syndrome have become intertwined and confused. While epilepsy is more common in ID and ASD than in typically developing children, ID and ASD are generally not caused by epilepsy. Seizures can make symptoms of ID and ASD worse and should be treated accordingly, but there is no evidence that normalizing the EEG with medications or even surgery will correct the language and other delays in these syndromes. This contrasts with children who have ESES in the setting of Landau-Kleffner syndrome, in whom treatment of the EEG may improve outcome and having the correct diagnosis is important.

Dravet Syndrome and the Generalized Epilepsy with Febrile Seizures Plus Spectrum

Dravet syndrome (DS), previously known as severe myoclonic epilepsy of infancy (SMEI), was first described in the late 1970s. It is now one of the most readily recognized of infantile epileptic encephalopathies because of its characteristic temperature-sensitive seizures and developmental course. It is quite rare, affecting an estimated 1:15,700 individuals in the United States. DS is most notable for onset of febrile seizures in the first year of life at the same time as, or shortly followed by, afebrile seizures and then developmental delays beginning in the second year of life. Often myoclonic seizures precede the first recognized febrile or nonfebrile tonic-clonic seizures but are not initially recognized. Compared to the benign simple febrile seizure described in Chapter 4, the febrile seizures seen in DS are typically prolonged (lasting 15 minutes or more) and often progress to status epilepticus. They are also more likely to be focal, with hemi-tonic-clonic (tonic-clonic seizures involving only half of the body) being a characteristic seizure type.

Along with more global developmental delays, unsteadiness in walking and behavioral problems can develop in the second year of life. Additionally, multiple seizure types, including myoclonus, atypical absence, tonic-clonic, and focal seizures, are frequent and difficult to treat during this period. After 5 years of age, seizures tend to decrease in frequency but remain difficult to treat in most cases. Delays in development continue, with a slowing in the achievement of milestones leading to bigger differences between these children and their typical peers, rather than regressions or loss of skills. Although there is a range of severity and seizure control improves somewhat in adults, it is rare for children to become seizure free, and there is typically some degree of cognitive, psychosocial, and movement difficulties in adulthood.

This epilepsy is genetically determined, and more than 80 percent of patients with DS have it because of a pathologic mutation in the SCN1A gene. In addition to understanding why your child has this particular type of epilepsy, getting this genetic diagnosis can help their physician determine treatment, as seizure drugs that block sodium channels may make seizures worse in DS. The SCN1A mutations that cause DS almost always arise spontaneously in children and are not inherited from parents, although there are some exceptions. Several other genes can cause DS, but these are much rarer and may not have the same implications for treatment.

It is important to recognize that, while the first seizure occurs in the setting of fever due to an infection or a vaccine, this does not mean that a specific infection or vaccination causes the syndrome. Rather, they are just the triggers that bring out the symptoms of the disorder. Avoiding fevers, infections, or vaccines may or may not delay symptoms temporarily but will not prevent the epilepsy syndrome altogether in a child that has a DS-causing gene mutation.

There are families in which multiple family members have febrile seizures and varying forms of nonfebrile seizures, suggesting inherited epilepsy. These families were characterized in the 1990s as having generalized epilepsy with febrile seizures plus (GEFS+). There is a range of characteristics in different families and even in different patients in the same family regarding type and prominence of nonfebrile seizures, typical versus atypical development, and outgrowing seizures or not, but all share the common association with febrile seizures. It is now recognized that SCN1A and other genes associated with DS can be the cause of epilepsy in these families. Interestingly, in contrast to most DS children, where the mutation causing the syndrome is spontaneous in the child, in these families, the mutations are inherited. This argues that there is spectrum between GEFS+ and DS, with genetic variants that cause milder forms of epilepsy on the GEFS+ end being more likely to be passed on through generations with varying degrees of symptoms. On the other end of this spectrum, the variants that cause DS typically cause such severe epilepsy syndromes that they do not get passed on to a next generation.

Neonatal Seizures

Seizures in a newborn can have many different causes. They occur in 1–3 per 1,000 live births in term infants and perhaps ten times more frequently in preterm newborns. They are often the consequence of lack of oxygen to the fetus before and rarely during labor, due to metabolic disorders, infections, stroke, or structural developmental disorders. Seizures in a newborn that are due to trauma, stroke, or difficulties with delivery may subside over the first days of life and may or may not lead to epilepsy later in life, but they are a sign that there was some degree of injury at the time.

Neonatal seizures can also be the result of genetic changes, with a wide range of outcomes. For example, benign familial neonatal-infantile seizures start within the first few days of life in a child who had a normal birth and delivery, and their course is characterized by seizures that can be treated with medication and normal development; eventually seizures are outgrown. Pyridoxine-dependent seizures are often characterized by seizures in utero, which the mother might describe as hiccups, and seizures starting immediately after birth. If 100 mg of pyridoxine (vitamin B6) is given, seizures usually stop almost immediately. If not recognized and treated appropriately, however, severe seizures that are not responsive to medication will persist. There are also multiple other genetic epilepsy syndromes that may present in the neonatal period and progress to severe and difficult-to-treat epileptic encephalopathies with associated cognitive and physical impairments regardless of what treatments are tried.

Unfortunately, it is not always possible to determine which end of the spectrum, from mild to severe, a child will fall into when they are first born. Because of the risk that a treatable infection, metabolic or vascular disorder, or structural problem could be causing seizures, even a neonate with a benign epilepsy syndrome may undergo extensive evaluations and treatments in a neonatal intensive care unit in the early days of life as a result of their often-severe seizures. This process can be more frightening than the ultimate outlook of self-limited seizures and typical development. In contrast, some neonates who have significant neurological dysfunction and will go on to have very severe epilepsy may appear relatively well in the days and weeks after birth. Communication regarding progress and changes, as well as follow-up with providers, is important to making sure that each child receives the appropriate evaluations and treatment.

CHAPTER 9

The Epilepsies of Childhood, Part II

Special Causes

When a child is diagnosed with epilepsy, the most common question that comes next is, "Why does my child have epilepsy?" Sometimes the answer to this question is readily apparent to the child's treatment team based on physical exam, EEG, imaging findings, or medical history. Sometimes an answer cannot be found after extensive investigations. In some cases, understanding what exactly caused a child's epilepsy may be helpful in guiding treatment. In other cases, searching for a definite cause may not be as helpful.

In certain situations, a child's doctor may not put them through extensive evaluations to find a cause. This may be because a specific cause is unlikely to be found or the benefits of finding an answer are unlikely to outweigh the burden of these tests, and not because they don't care about the child or finding important answers. In addition to the question of why a child has epilepsy, many parents' next question is, "Did I do something wrong?" While each child is unique, the vast majority of childhood epilepsies cannot be prevented by anyone. Knowing more about some of the possible causes of epilepsy, in general, can be helpful to understanding why this is the case.

Just as epilepsy has many forms, it has many causes as well. In general, these can be divided into epilepsy that is the result of an injury to the brain and epilepsy that is due to a change in the way the brain develops, typically from known or unknown genetic factors. Within each of these categories, there are more or less severe injuries or dramatic changes that may have more or less of an effect on the overall function of the brain for varying periods. Common causes of injury that can lead to epilepsy include stroke, head trauma, lack of oxygen, bleeding in the brain, tumors, infections, and immune system dysfunction. Injuries at any time in development, either before or after birth, can predispose children to epilepsy. Injuries that occur early in brain development may also change the way the brain develops, creating an additional risk for epilepsy. Most data indicate that about a quarter to a third of epilepsies occur as a result of the different types of injury or external factors, but most changes that result in epilepsy are either genetically determined or *idiopathic*. As we learn more, we are finding that those "idiopathic" cases are also likely genetic but involve mechanisms that we do not yet fully understand. This has led to the International League Against Epilepsy (ILAE) to categorize many epilepsies as *genetic generalized epilepsies* regardless of whether there is a known genetic cause.

In any discussion of childhood epilepsy and its causes, it is important to note that just as there is variability in the severity of seizures and the response to treatment within each epilepsy syndrome, there is also variability in the association of the seizures with other differences in neurological development. Most children who have epilepsy do not have intellectual disability (ID), autism spectrum disorder (ASD), cerebral palsy, or other neurological or medical problems. Most children who do have ID, ASD, or cerebral palsy do not have epilepsy. Nonetheless, sometimes brain damage due to lack of oxygen, strokes, head trauma, or genetically determined changes in brain development may lead to epilepsy as well as to ID, ASD, cerebral palsy, or other neurological problems.

Some important causes of epilepsy are discussed in more detail below, but this discussion does not include all the specific causes of epilepsy for each unique child. Additionally, particularly in the more "benign" forms of epilepsy, where seizures respond to medications and children eventually outgrow the seizures, a specific cause may not always be found.

Acquired Conditions that Cause Epilepsy

Strokes

Surprising as it may seem, strokes are not uncommon in the newborn period. Thrombosis (blockage) of one or more arteries may occur in the days before or after birth, resulting in a stroke. Often such strokes are difficult to detect because most of the infant's movements are not willful, cortical movements. Occasionally the strokes are heralded by seizures in the newborn, but often the only sign of a stroke is that the child displays left-handedness or right-handedness at an age when children should not have a dominant side. The infant splashing in the bath may use only one arm. As the infant begins to sit, they may avoid using one arm to prop themselves up. It looks like a preference for one side, but this kind of preference should not be seen in a young baby. Walking may be delayed because of the weakness or spasticity of one leg. Even the handedness may go unnoticed for many months. Only when the infant has a seizure and is carefully examined, or has imaging of the brain because of the seizure, is the stroke diagnosed. The scan shows an absence of brain tissue in the area to which the blood supply was blocked that may be surrounded by scarring. Seizures may result from abnormally functioning cells in a scar or at the edge of where tissue was lost or from abnormalities in the way the brain functions as a network due to the loss of those cells that were reabsorbed, leaving behind only fluid.

These children are usually of normal intelligence. Some, but not all, develop seizures on the weak side of the body. If the seizures are difficult to control with medication, and if the child is already paralyzed on that side, surgical removal of the damaged cortex might be appropriate.

This could involve a hemispherectomy (removal of that side of the brain—see Chapter 14) or removal of a smaller portion of the brain that is affected. Either may help the child to become seizure free, medication free, and able to lead a more normal life.

Strokes need not always affect a major artery but may sometimes affect only small branches of an artery, and the result is local scarring, which may cause epilepsy. Abnormalities of blood vessels called *arterio-*

venous malformations or blockage of veins within the brain may have similar effects.

Infections

Acute bacterial and viral infections of the brain (meningitis and encephalitis) may cause acute seizures and may occasionally damage the brain and result in epilepsy. Infections that occur before birth may also damage the brain and lead to epilepsy. We are fortunate that several very severe bacterial infections that used to cause seizures can now be prevented with vaccines: H. influenza, meningococcal, and pneumonia. They can be devastating, and vaccination is critical in preventing them. One of the most common infections of the brain worldwide is cysticercosis; in some countries, this may be the most common cause of epilepsy, but in the United States, it is a rare cause of seizures. A doctor will suspect this diagnosis when single or multiple areas of typical calcification, the result of cysts within the brain, are spotted on a CT or MRI scan.

Another brain infection is toxoplasmosis, an infection spread by underprocessed food and, in some parts of the world, cats. If a pregnant woman acquires this infection, it may be transmitted to her baby and cause scarring in the brain. Infection, often undetectable in the newborn, may first be manifested as intellectual disability or as seizures. An MRI scan can detect scars within the brain and aid in diagnosis. Also, small scars on the retina in the back of the eye may be noted by your child's physician and suggest a diagnosis. In addition, blood tests can confirm what the observations suggest. Suspected toxoplasmosis is often treated in an attempt to prevent further damage. The treatment of seizures in affected children is similar to the treatment for those in other forms of epilepsy.

Herpes simplex virus (HSV) is an extremely common human infection. In rare cases it can spread to the brain and have devastating effects. It takes two forms. One is the cold sore that occurs around the mouth, and the other is genital lesions. A baby born to a woman whose cervix is actively infected with HSV may, in turn, acquire the virus during delivery, which may devastate the child's brain, producing severe intellectual disability, cerebral palsy, and epilepsy. In addition, a brain infection caused by oral HSV may be acquired at any age and produce focal seizures and an overwhelming encephalitis. Early detection may enable treatment to be more effective. Children who survive have variable degrees of brain damage and epilepsy.

In addition to toxoplasmosis and herpes simplex virus, multiple congenital infections (infections occurring during fetal development) can lead to multiple organ problems as well as varying forms of brain injury, epilepsy, and often intellectual disability. These are often referred to as the TORCH infections, so named after the most notable individual causes (toxoplasmosis, other, rubella, cytomegalovirus, and herpes simplex virus). Multiple infections can be included in the *other* category, many of which cannot be specifically identified in an individual child. Some are very rare, but the profound effect on brain development makes them more likely to be identified. This includes the mosquito-borne Zika virus, which drew a lot of media attention in 2015 and 2016 when large outbreaks occurred in the Americas, causing prominent microcephaly; almost 70 percent prevalence of epilepsy was associated with infants whose mothers were infected during pregnancy. Fortunately, the number of Zika virus infections declined rapidly in 2017.

Human immunodeficiency virus (HIV), the virus that causes acquired immunodeficiency syndrome (AIDS), is less commonly transmitted to infants born to mothers infected with HIV than it was in the past. This is predominately the result of better HIV treatments, as infection of the infant may be preventable by treating the mother prior to or at the time of delivery. With current drug regimens and treatments as well as screening of all pregnant women for the virus, the number of children infected by their mothers has plummeted in the last 20 years. When the virus does affect the child during pregnancy or delivery, however, it can produce seizures. The multiple infections that are byproducts of the immunosuppression due to HIV infection may also affect the brain and cause seizures. Secondary infections require specific treatment, but the seizures are often treated with standard antiseizure medication.

Other viral causes of meningitis include arboviruses such as West Nile, dengue, chikungunya, and Japanese encephalitis. These are mosquito borne and occur in various parts of the world.

Autoimmune Disorders

A rare form of progressive unilateral seizures, usually associated with a progressive hemiparesis (weakness of one side of the body), has been termed Rasmussen's syndrome after the Canadian neurosurgeon who first described it. The sudden onset of intense, constant focal seizures may indicate the presence of Rasmussen's syndrome, a focal, unilateral encephalitis-like condition. While sometimes beginning with either a generalized or a unilateral tonic-clonic seizure, this condition frequently involves a state called *epilepsia partialis continua* (continuous focal epilepsy). The hand, face, or foot may jerk continuously. This condition is uniformly progressive, spreading to seemingly random places throughout the involved hemisphere.

Although Rasmussen's syndrome was originally thought to be viral in origin, and more recent studies suggest that it is autoimmune (the body's immune system attacking the brain) in nature, a definite cause is not completely understood. The seizures do not respond to any current antiseizure medications. Steroids have sometimes had a transient beneficial effect, as has plasmapheresis (washing the blood plasma to remove the antibodies), the administration of large doses of intravenous gamma globulin, or chronic immune-suppressing medications. All these therapies give temporary relief at best from the unstoppable progression of this condition and come with associated risks.

Until some more effective form of immunotherapy becomes available, the only effective treatment is hemispheric disconnection (surgically disconnecting the affected side of the brain from the rest of the brain). Removal or disconnection of only portions of the affected side always results in recurrence of the seizures in the remaining portions. This peculiar condition is limited to one half of the brain. Therefore, disconnection of the affected half, if done early in the course of the disease, results in cessation of the seizures and allows more normal intellectual development. After surgery there will be paralysis of one side of the body and loss of vision to that side, but these children walk, run, and go to school. Without surgery, the outcomes are worse.

Rasmussen's syndrome is thought to be part of the larger category of autoimmune-related epilepsies, where the body's immune system attacks a particular part of the brain. Although more common in adults, in recent years the contribution of autoimmune disorders to epilepsy in children and adolescence has been increasingly recognized and researched. Of note is NMDA receptor antibody encephalitis, which results from the immune system creating antibodies that target the NMDA receptor in the brain. The NMDA receptor is a major protein in the brain that is important in learning and memory, and when patients have an autoantibody toward this protein, a syndrome of severely altered behavior, cognition, abnormal movements, and seizures results.

In some cases, a tumor called a teratoma can be found in the ovaries as the cause of this syndrome, but in other cases, no cause can be found. It is diagnosed based on clinical symptoms and the presence of antibodies in the blood or spinal fluid. As opposed to Rasmussen's encephalitis, where only one hemisphere is affected, brain surgery is not generally considered a treatment, and immune system–modulating treatments, as well as removing the tumor if present, are the primary therapies.

Genetic Conditions that Cause Epilepsy

The development of the brain includes a series of events in which cells move and interconnections are established in a process so complex that it amazes and awes physicians. This process is controlled by the coordinated turning on and off of genes in different cells at different times, the ability of cells to send and receive signals telling them where to go and when and what types of proteins that they express on their cell surface. Many different abnormalities can occur during brain development as a result of either a change in one or many genes or external factors. As a result, the cells may be too large, misconnected, or malformed. They may not move to the proper place in the brain, or they may express too much or too little of a protein that is needed to control the excitability and proper functioning of brain cells.

On occasion, these abnormalities may be focal and produce focal seizures or focal motor deficits. The latter may be surgically treated if that area of the brain can be safely removed. This is determined during a surgical evaluation (Chapter 14). Less commonly, these developmental abnormalities may involve severe and extensive changes to only one half of the brain, resulting in paralysis of one side of the body and uni-lateral seizures. If with such abnormalities, a child has uncontrollable seizures, disconnection of that abnormal half of the brain (functional hemispherectomy) may be a lifesaving and seizure-curing procedure (Chapter 14).

Developmental changes that involve the entire brain are less likely to be treated with surgeries to remove parts of the brain, and depend-ing on the type of changes, different types of medications or alternative treatments may be more effective. As with focal developmental changes, those that affect the entire brain can have a wide range of severity. This can be seen in genetic changes that alter the expression of ion chan-nels (cell surface proteins that control electrical excitability of neurons, the primary electrical cells of the brain). On the milder end of epilepsy severity, genetic changes in ion channel genes may result in increased risk of seizures and treatment-responsive epilepsy that is present only in certain periods of development. These children's brains may appear structurally normal, and they may have typical cognitive development.

On the more severe end, other ion channel abnormalities can pro-duce severe epilepsy that is lifelong. In addition, changes in other types of genes may result in significant changes in the number and migration of cells early in brain development, resulting in large changes in brain structure and significant lifelong epilepsy that may be difficult to treat. Such severe abnormalities in brain development involving the entire brain are more likely to be accompanied by ID and cerebral palsy, and changes in brain structure are more likely to show up on MRI. While the number of genetic changes that can result in epilepsy are too numerous to discuss in detail here, we briefly discuss how genetic changes can alter brain function, approaches to genetic evaluations, and some of the more common and well-known genetic changes.

How Do Genetic Changes Result in Epilepsy?

All the information required for human development is contained in each person's genetic information. It's important to have a basic un-derstanding of how this works to appreciate what your child's doctor is thinking about if they order genetic testing for your child. The genetic information is encoded by sequences of deoxyribonucleic acids, or DNA. Specific sequences of DNA make up individual genes that, in turn, code for proteins, which make up the structure and functioning components of our cells. In addition to the DNA that makes up our genes, there is also DNA in between and within genes that does not make protein but is required to organize the genes and regulate gene expression (whether a gene is turned on to make protein or is turned off). Despite the fact that each DNA molecule is submicroscopic, the number of DNA molecules in each cell is so numerous that if we were to stretch it all out like a string, it would be approximately 6 feet long—in a single cell.

All the DNA within a cell is folded and compacted into discrete chromosomes, however, with only small portions of the DNA being unfolded at a time to make proteins or to copy DNA for cell replication. Humans have 46 chromosomes that are arranged in 22 pairs of somatic (chromosomes common to everyone) and 1 pair of sex chromosomes that are the same in females (XX) and different in males (XY). Except for the male XY pair, each chromosome pair has two copies, or *alleles*, of every gene, with one chromosome inherited from a mother and one inherited from a father.

DNA can be changed and cause a change in the way that the brain develops and functions in many ways. An entire chromosome and all its genetic content can be deleted (too little DNA) or duplicated (too much DNA). This is what happens in the case of Down syndrome, otherwise known as trisomy 21, due to three copies of chromosome 21 being present instead of the typical two. These changes are usually diagnosed with a karyotype (a photograph of the chromosomes that are examined under a regular microscope) and often affect multiple organ systems, including the brain. Depending on which chromosome is affected, entire chromosome deletion or duplication may result in death in utero or shortly after birth.

Smaller pieces of chromosomes can also be deleted or duplicated. Because these changes affect a smaller number of genes, they may result in less severe changes, depending on what genes are affected, than when the entire chromosome is involved. Duplications or deletions of parts of chromosomes are referred to as copy number variations (CNVs) and can be diagnosed either by a karyotype, when very large, or by a chromosomal microarray. These are much more sophisticated biochemical techniques that allow changes to be measured at a much more detailed level than a karyotype. Depending on what genetic problem your doctor is looking for, different microarrays might be ordered. Chromosomal CNVs are thought to account for up to 10 percent of patients with genetic epilepsy but may be more common in children who also have intellectual disability, autism, or psychiatric problems.

Changes within DNA sequences or deletions or duplications of single genes can also cause epilepsy. Changes within the DNA sequence can be thought of as changing the spelling of a word. Sometimes a substitution is made that still allows the meaning of the word to be understood. Similarly, some DNA changes don't change gene function significantly. Sometimes spelling substitutions are made that result in changing the meaning of a word or in a nonsensical word. Similarly, some DNA changes result in a gene that encodes for a nonfunctional protein, a protein with altered levels of function, or a protein that is recognized as abnormal by other cellular machinery and is therefore destroyed. A single gene can be deleted or duplicated, resulting in too much or too little protein.

Changes in the gene sequence can be detected by sequencing of the gene that is thought to be altered; alternatively, we can sequence large numbers of genes that are thought to be involved in genetic epilepsy. This is referred to as a *gene panel*. We can also sequence all an individual's genes with whole exome sequencing (WES). Because of the large amounts of data that WES generates, however, there is significant cost and data analysis involved, and the results should be interpreted by specialists. Sometimes changes from the "typical," or reference, DNA are noted, but even experts don't understand what, if any, biological change may have happened because of it, so they can't tell you if it is an important finding for your child. Additionally, because WES does not examine the DNA that does not code for a gene or protein, a negative test does not completely exclude a genetic cause.

Spontaneous and Inherited Genetic Changes

In all these cases, if the gene (or group of genes) that is changed is important for brain development and function, the change can result in neurological symptoms including epilepsy. In some cases, a genetic change in only one of the two gene copies (alleles) is enough to cause a problem. We refer to these as *autosomal dominant disorders*. In these disorders, genetic changes often arise spontaneously (*de novo*) only in the affected child and are not inherited. If they are inherited, they are inherited from only one parent, and that parent typically, but not always, has similar symptoms. For example, benign familial neonatal-infantile epilepsy is most commonly caused by a sequence change in one copy of the KCNQ2 gene that encodes a potassium ion channel. The resulting dysfunction results in altered cellular excitability and seizures beginning in the neonatal period. Although patients typically outgrow seizures in early childhood, they have a 50 percent chance of passing the abnormal gene on to their children, and each child with the abnormal gene will have similar seizures when very young.

In many cases both copies of a gene have to be altered to create a problem with brain function. If inherited, this means that both parents have to give an abnormal gene to the child. When this happens, parents typically have only one abnormal copy of the gene and are not affected. Although parents each have a 50 percent chance of passing an abnormal gene to their child, because both parents have to give the abnormal copy, each child has only a 25 percent chance of being affected. Each child has a 50 percent chance of being a carrier, having one abnormal copy, like their parents. Often these autosomal recessive disorders are more severe than the autosomal dominant epilepsy disorders.

For example, in the previous chapter we discussed that certain children could have very severe seizures at birth or before birth that are responsive to treatment with vitamin B6. This pyridoxal 5'-phosphate (B6)-dependent epilepsy is an autosomal recessive epilepsy caused by a child inheriting an abnormal copy of the PNPO gene from each parent. This gene encodes an enzyme required for metabolism of B6 from food to a form that can be used by the body and that is necessary for normal production of neurotransmitters. Without any functional enzyme, the child does not have the ability to metabolize B6. Because parents have only one abnormal copy, they have enough enzyme and do not have epilepsy and the other symptoms associated with this disorder.

In addition to autosomal dominant and autosomal recessive genetic disorders, if a particular epilepsy-causing gene is present on one of the sex-specific chromosomes, there may be sex-specific patterns of symptoms in children. Typical females carry two X chromosomes, and typical males have one X chromosome and a unique Y chromosome. This difference means that females have two copies of many genes that males have only one copy of, and males have some genes that females do not have because they have a Y chromosome. While the actual ability of genes to be expressed is tightly regulated, and one copy of the X chromosome is "turned off" in each cell of a female, this means that certain disorders may affect males or females more.

For example, Rett syndrome is a severe disorder characterized by progressive autistic regression after approximately 18 months of age, microcephaly, intellectual disability, cerebral palsy, and severe epilepsy that typically occurs only in girls because the MECP2 gene that causes the disorder is on the X chromosome. This gene is so important to brain development that when a boy's only copy is dysfunctional, he does not survive embryonic development. Because the abnormal copy may be the "turned on" copy in only a portion of the cells in females, they survive but are severely affected. In the case of fragile X syndrome, changes in the FMRP gene, which is also on the X chromosome, results in intellectual disability and possibly autism and epilepsy in males who inherit it from their mothers, but females can carry the abnormal copy of the gene and pass it on with much milder and often different symptoms.

Who Should Be Tested for Genetic Causes of Epilepsy?

Genetic causes of epilepsy are common and should always be considered, but testing for this is not absolutely necessary in every case. An investigation into genetic causes should be considered when epilepsy is severe and does not respond to medications. This is even more important if severe epilepsy starts before the age of 2 years. It should also be considered when there is an association with intellectual disability, autism, or other congenital changes in other organ systems that may suggest a more globally atypical development of the brain. Additionally, it should be considered when there is a distinct family history of multiple members with epilepsy with or without other neurological changes that may suggest inherited genetic changes.

Potential Risks and Benefits of Evaluating for a Genetic Cause

Our understanding of the genetics of epilepsy is rapidly expanding. Given advances in technology and the ability to screen all of a patient's genes with a single test using techniques such as chromosomal microarrays and whole exome sequencing, our understanding will continue to expand. Yet, with this abundance of information comes a need for careful interpretation and proper counseling. Changes that arise only in the affected child can be passed on by that child only if they have children. Changes that are the result of genes inherited from one or both parents have implications for parents, siblings, and the children of siblings as well. Broad testing such as WES and microarrays may also reveal information about other disease processes not related to the nervous system, with potential implications for both child and family. For this reason, when a genetic change is suspected, investigations should be undertaken with physicians and genetic counselors who are able to interpret the information that is available.

Each patient will have specific needs when it comes to genetic counseling, but everyone should be aware of some general principles about genetic testing for epilepsy. The first is that there are multiple possible results for any testing strategy. At a minimum, there is the possibility that results will lead to a diagnosis, that results will be negative, or that results will be uncertain.

For patients who receive a diagnosis, there are also many possibilities. The diagnosis may or may not lead to a change in symptomatic treatments or let the child's provider know to avoid certain medications or treatments. Results may indicate that other tests need to be undertaken to look for changes in other organ systems that may not have been considered to be affected previously. It is rare that obtaining a genetic diagnosis leads to a disease-modifying treatment or cure, although exceptions are increasing every day as scientific advances are made. Some examples include metabolic disorders in which children lack an enzyme important for energy metabolism of cells, resulting in energy failure. Knowing what gene and corresponding enzyme is not functioning correctly can inform about specific diets or supplements, as described for pyridoxine-dependent epilepsy in Chapter 8 and earlier in this chapter.

In addition, Glut1-deficiency syndrome results from mutations in the SLC2A1 gene. This gene encodes for the glucose transporter type 1 (Glut1), which brings glucose across the blood-brain barrier to be used by all brain cells for energy. With absence or dysfunction of this transporter, there is energy depletion, resulting in epilepsy and varying degrees of microcephaly (small head size), intellectual disability, and movement disorders. Treatment with the ketogenic diet, which provides ketones as alternates to glucose as the major energy source (see Chapter 12), may modify the course of this syndrome.

While disease-altering changes in treatments because of a genetic diagnosis are relatively rare, the most common benefit is a better understanding of prognosis. This may allow families to prepare for unexpected changes in the future and optimize interventions. It is important to understand that in certain cases, a dire prognosis may be given and cannot be changed. Finally, for many, a genetic diagnosis may benefit the child and family merely by ending the diagnostic odyssey, enabling them to simply know why and possibly what to expect.

Not receiving a diagnosis is often frustrating. The absence of a diagnosis may mean that there is not a genetic cause or that the genetic cause cannot be detected with current technology. Testing may also detect changes in genes with unclear information as to whether these changes are responsible for epilepsy. The change may be in a gene that has never been reported as associated with epilepsy but is suspected to be involved in brain development, or it can be in a known epilepsy gene but whether the change is enough to alter the function of the gene may be unclear. This is referred to as a variant of uncertain significance. Negative results or variants of uncertain significance can be the most frustrating outcome for families and providers, but the testing can be revisited at intervals, usually of one to two years, to see if changes in knowledge or technology affect interpretation of results or detect more definitive changes.

Specific Genetic Syndromes
Some specific genetic causes of epilepsy have already been discussed in Chapter 8 and earlier in this chapter. While it is not possible to discuss the hundreds of genes and genetic syndromes within this book, some specific genetic syndromes deserve specific mention and detailed discussion.

The Neurocutaneous Syndromes
As discussed above, atypical cellular development sometimes leads to changes in the brain that affect epilepsy and cognitive development. Some of these genetic changes also result in abnormal development of skin and other organs. Within this category are many genetic causes and syndromes, but some of the most recognizable and well understood are the neurocutaneous syndromes (involving the brain and the skin) tuberous sclerosis and Sturge-Weber syndrome.

Tuberous Sclerosis
Tuberous sclerosis complex (TSC) is an inherited or *de novo* genetic condition in which children may have an abnormality of cell development affecting many organs of the body. In the brain, abnormal cells may form nonmalignant tumors known as hamartomas. These occur within the brain tissue, where they are called *tubers*, and in the linings of the ventricles (fluid-filled spaces of the brain), where they are called *subependymal nodules*. Tumors and other lesions can also occur in the kidney, heart, eyes, and skin. The most common finding that triggers an evaluation for the diagnosis of tuberous sclerosis is multiple white spots that appear on the skin (Figure 9.1). The CT or MRI scan may show the tubers or areas of calcification. Older children may develop acne-like changes on their faces. In addition, a constellation of findings on the nails, heart, and kidneys may suggest the diagnosis. Genetic testing typically confirms the diagnosis with mutations in either the TSC1 or TSC2 gene. These two genes are part of a protein complex that reg-

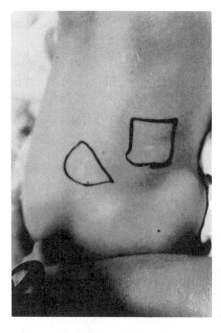

FIGURE 9.1. Tuberous sclerosis.
Multiple white spots, subtle and
ash-leaf shaped, are symptomatic.

ulates cell growth and division, and loss of their function results in abnormal cell growth. The cellular abnormalities and hamartomas may in turn cause epilepsy, either focal or generalized. Children with tuberous sclerosis can also develop infantile spasms and Lennox-Gastaut syndrome (Chapter 8).

The outcome of children with tuberous sclerosis varies, as does their epilepsy. Some individuals may be of normal intelligence with no significant disability. Others may have substantial ID and difficult-to-control seizures. Early awareness of this diagnosis is important for several reasons. Although the tubers and subependymal nodules are not malignant, they can cause problems based on size and location and need to be monitored. Similarly, associated kidney and cardiac changes may need to be addressed. Awareness of the diagnosis may also affect medication choice. Everolimus is a disease-specific and potentially disease-modifying drug that targets the molecular pathway that is abnormal in TSC. Long-term treatment may improve seizures as well as control TSC tumors, subependymal giant cell astrocytoma, and renal angiomyolipoma. Additionally, for infants who develop infantile spasms as a result of TSC, first-line treatment is typically vigabatrin rather than the standard steroid treatments used first in other causes.

Although there are usually many tuberous lesions within the brain, sometimes only one of them is causing the seizures. Therefore, if a child with tuberous sclerosis has difficult-to-control seizures, it may be worth seeing a pediatric epileptologist at an epilepsy center that does sophisticated epilepsy monitoring and surgery to assess if the child might be a candidate for surgery.

Sturge-Weber Syndrome

Sturge-Weber syndrome (SWS) is caused by a developmental abnormality of the blood vessels to the face and the developing brain. The underlying genetic cause is a somatic mutation in the GNAQ gene, which makes a protein important in regulating blood vessels. Somatic mutations are those that occur in the cells of an embryo *after* fertilization and the first cell divisions. This means that not all cells in the body have the mutation and that the mutation is not inherited from parents. It also means that there is variability in the severity and presentation of SWS depending on what and how many cells carry the mutant copy of the gene verses the normal copy. No one knows how or why this mutation occurs.

Children with SWS almost always have a "port-wine stain" (Figure 9.2), also called an *angioma*. This angioma always involves the forehead and the area around an eye (first division of the facial nerve) but may also involve the rest of the face on one or both sides. The port-wine stain can produce a cosmetic handicap, and the child should be seen by a dermatologist in early infancy. Laser technology has enabled the removal of most traces of the stain with minimal scarring. Results are better with earlier treatment.

In addition to the facial birthmark, children with SWS may have seizures, a progressive hemiparesis (weakness on one side of the body), developmental delay, and glaucoma (increased pressure in the eye, which may lead to blindness). Glaucoma occurs in more than half of children with SWS and usually starts in the first year of life. It is treatable. All children with SWS should be seen by an ophthalmologist and followed periodically throughout their life.

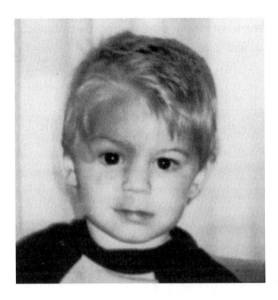

FIGURE 9.2. Sturge-Weber syndrome. Note the birthmark over the child's right forehead, eye, and lip.

The vascular abnormality involves the coverings of the brain as well as the face and results in seizures in 80 percent of cases and in a paralysis of the opposite side of the body in 65 percent. Seizures occur in more than 80 percent of children with SWS, the majority beginning during the first year of life. One-quarter of the children achieve full seizure control with medication, one-half achieve partial seizure control, and one-quarter report no seizure control with medication. Early onset seizures are the most difficult to control. There is also a correlation between the age of seizure onset and motor development and IQ. Children whose onset of seizures occur within the first year and whose seizures are not controlled have a higher risk of subnormal development. Normal intelligence was found in 44 percent of all individuals with SWS and in 33 percent of those with seizures. Hemispherectomy, or removal of the affected part of the brain, has been done in infants and children with SWS whose seizures were difficult to control; the ideal timing of the surgery remains a matter of debate.

Degenerative Diseases

Several progressive, degenerative diseases of the brain affect children. Epilepsy is commonly seen in most of them. One group is called storage diseases, because the proteins and fats that are normally broken down to waste products (metabolized) and eliminated from the body cannot be broken down in these rare inherited metabolic conditions. Waste products accumulate within nerve cells and affect their function, leading to epilepsy and intellectual disability. These progressive conditions are typically due to a change in one of the genes involved in the particular metabolic pathway. They may be fatal, but the duration of the illness may be quite variable, and there may be specific treatments depending on the disorder.

Among these conditions are Tay-Sachs disease (GM2 gangliosidosis), Batten's disease (ceroid lipofuscinosis), and the various leukodystrophies. Many other diseases affect metabolism of brain cells and result in epilepsy as well as deterioration of intellect and/or motor function. Each of these has its own age of onset, its own course, and its own outcome. It is beyond the scope of this book to discuss them individually, but some that were previously untreatable now have life-extending treatments.

Although many of the epilepsy syndromes and some of these infections sound very frightening and can be devastating to both the child and the family, fortunately these conditions are uncommon, as are the degenerative diseases. Most children with epilepsy do not have these conditions, and their seizures are controlled. Most children with epilepsy do very well.

PART III

Treatment

CHAPTER 10

Using Medicines

Philosophy of Treatment

Although it was once believed that all seizures should be treated, just because they were there, now it is generally believed that no judgment can cover every individual. Decisions about treatment should be made by the patient (or parent) *and* the physician, acting in partnership. The decision should be based on risk-benefit analysis.

• The risks and consequences of each medication vary with the medicine, the dose, the individual's reaction to the medicine, the age of the child, and the length of time the child takes the medicine.

• The risk of further seizures varies markedly with the type of seizure, the frequency of seizures, and even the time of day in which they occur. A child who has only occasional tonic-clonic seizures at night will face very different risks from a child whose seizures occur during the day. A child with occasional focal seizures with impaired awareness has different risks from the child with tonic-clonic seizures or the child with frequent absence seizures.

Most people's seizures can be controlled with a single medicine used in a proper dose to achieve a proper blood level for that individual. *There is no "correct" dose of a given medication.* The "proper" dose of medication is the dose that completely controls the seizures without causing significant side effects. *There is not a "correct" medication as such. Some medicines work better for some types of seizures than for others. The correct medicine is the one that works.*

The treatment of epilepsy is empirical. This means that the treatment of each person's seizures is a trial or search to find the appropriate dose of the best medicine for that individual. This "experimentation" is often frustrating to parents, since they are used to physicians' knowing, for example, the right antibiotic and dose to use for a child's ear infection. For antibiotics, we know the function, the proper dose, and the side effects. We know how much is necessary to kill the bacteria causing the infection. We can test the drug's effectiveness in the laboratory. We also know, for example, how "heart drugs" work and their side effects; we can use the electrocardiogram (EKG) to see if they are working or if they are producing toxicity. But, since we do not fully understand how anti-seizure medications work, and since we do not understand the factors that permit a seizure to occur at a specific time, each child must be his own "laboratory" as a doctor attempts to find the proper dose of the best medication. Side effects will vary with each child's metabolism and their individual reaction to the medication.

Terms You Need to Know

Medication, or Drug, Levels

The term *drug level* refers to the amount of a medication in the blood—to be more precise, the serum levels, since the medication is in the liquid portion of your blood (serum) rather than in the red blood cells. When we measure drug levels or blood levels, we usually measure the total amount of a medication in the serum.

Toxicity

The term *toxicity* covers a multitude of things. Toxicity, in general, refers to all the adverse (bad) effects of a medication. There are two major forms of such toxicity, allergic and dose related.

Allergic reactions are idiosyncratic, which means that each person is different and may react in an unusual fashion to the medication. While anyone may have an allergic reaction to any medication, some medications are more likely to produce reactions than others. Allergic reactions may be mild (a slight rash) or severe (if the rash continues to spread and involves the membranes of the mouth). Such a severe reaction, termed the Stevens-Johnson syndrome, may even be fatal. Allergic rashes to drugs usually occur within the first three to four weeks after starting the medication. We warn every patient starting a new medicine:

Notify your physician immediately if a rash appears and stop taking the medication until you are seen by the physician.

Most rashes are the result of viruses, bites, or allergies to something else, but it is always better to be safe.

Other types of allergic or idiosyncratic reactions can involve the liver, pancreas, bone marrow, or blood cells. They may be mild, severe, or even fatal. Some physicians obtain blood chemistries and liver function tests before starting a new medication as a baseline against which to measure any changes that may occur. They repeat the tests periodically. Others feel that these reactions are very rare and tell families that if the child is tired, weak, jaundiced (has yellowness of the eyes), loses appetite, or begins to bruise easily or to bleed, these could be signs of reactions to the medications. It is always wise to question a new medication if your child is less well in any way after having started it. The physician should be notified if any of these symptoms appears, and the medication should be stopped until the cause is found. Whether one of these approaches is more successful than the other at recognizing the early signs of systemic reactions and at preventing serious consequences is unclear.

Dose-related toxicity depends on the amount of the medication in the brain. It may display itself as sedation (sleepiness), ataxia (unsteadiness), tremor, or even increasing problems with learning. Dose-related toxicities are important to recognize and when recognized are seldom serious because they are reversible by decreasing or discontinuing the drug.

Half-Life

The half-life is the amount of time it takes for one half of the medication in the body to be metabolized (broken down) or excreted. Therefore, if a dose of a medicine reaches a level of 10 in your body, that drug's half-life is the amount of time it takes until the blood level decreases to 5 (see Figure 10.1). This is important to you because the half-life for some medicines is only a few hours, but for others it may be days. A medication's half-life will determine how often your child must take their medicine—one, two, or, rarely, four times per day. The half-life varies with each medication and with the age of the child.

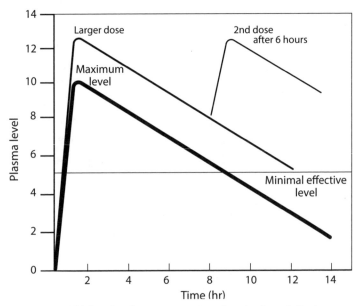

FIGURE 10.1. Half-life of a drug. Drugs are absorbed at different rates. The drug taken by mouth takes approximately an hour to reach its maximum blood (plasma) level of 10, then is slowly metabolized and excreted. The amount in the blood falls to half of its maximum level (5) 8 hours later; thus, the half-life of this drug is 8 hours. If a second dose were to be given 6 hours after the first, the body would be absorbing new medicine, and the blood level would never fall below the minimum effective level for preventing seizures.

We must allow each new medication sufficient time before we know whether it is going to work. For example, since ethosuximide (Zarontin) has a half-life of about 30 hours in a child, it will take at least 5 days to achieve a steady state. If your child is still having absence seizures 3 days after starting ethosuximide, or after increasing the dose, it may not mean that the medication will not work. It may mean, rather, that there hasn't been enough time to test that dose of the medicine. You have to be patient.

Q. *"My child has failed four medications in the past three weeks. What do we do now?"*
A. You will probably need to stop, regroup, and maybe even start over again. None of the medications was given a sufficient trial to declare them a failure. None had sufficient time to reach a steady state, to determine if they could be effective. Trying to achieve seizure control quickly is the most frequent mistake we see. Individuals are given too many medications in too short a period. Patience on the part of the parent and the physician will, in the long run, pay off, and you will not discard medicines that might have worked. Each medication should be given approximately two weeks to reach steady state and several weeks to demonstrate effectiveness. If it then seems not to be working, the medication should be gradually increased to effectiveness or to toxicity before declaring it a failure and starting a new one. It may take two or three months before you can determine if medicine is effective.

Q. *"Sam takes his medicine three times each day but often forgets to take his after-school dose. What can I do about it?"*
A. Change his medication schedule. Most patients at least occasionally forget to take a dose of medication, and the more frequent the doses are, the more likely one is to forget.

• Individuals taking medicine once a day have been found to miss 10 percent of the doses. They may remember and take it late, but they usually remember.

• Individuals taking medicine twice a day on average miss 20 percent of the doses. Again, missed doses may be taken late.

• Individuals taking medicine three times a day forget 40 percent of the doses, and those taking medication four times a day miss even more.

There is virtually no reason to take medicine more than twice a day. Independent of the half-life, the steady state will almost always provide enough safety to permit twice-a-day dosing. Few medicines have such a small margin that they have dose-related toxicity when given twice a day. You can usually just give them at breakfast and dinnertime to make life easier; they don't usually have to be 12 hours apart exactly.

• *If* the medication is given twice a day, *and* the patient has seizures before the second dose, *then* you may want to give the medication three times a day or try another medication.

• *If* the medication is given twice a day, *and* the patient has signs of drug-related toxicity one to two hours after the dose, *then* their blood level at that time may be too high, and the physician may either reduce the dose, spread it out to three times each day, or change to another medicine.

Some medications are now made in a slow-release form. They are slowly absorbed and achieve a steadier state with fewer peaks and valleys. Evidence that they have less toxicity or greater efficacy is not strong.

Q. *"What will happen if my child forgets to take a dose of medication? What should we do?"*
A. Again, your child's steady-state blood level should be sufficiently consistent that forgetting a single dose should make little difference. They should take the missed dose when they remember. Missing repeated doses is a different matter; that may affect your child's seizure control. It is often difficult to remember whether you actually took your medicine or if you only thought that you took it. A daily pillbox (some with several sections for separate doses) enables you and your child to check to see if the pills have been consumed or if they are still in the box.

Medication adherence (remembering to take medicine routinely as prescribed) is a problem for many people who have to take medicine on a chronic, daily basis. Lack of adherence can be caused by various factors, including the patient or family not understanding enough about the medication and how it works. It can also be caused by patients and families not being able to afford it on a regular basis. Help is available from various sources, and they need to be utilized. These include medication managers through a health care plan, the Health Resources and Services Administration (www.hrsa.gov), and the pharmaceutical company involved. These are issues that need to be discussed openly. Suggestions also include simplifying the regimen as much as possible, taking the medicine at the same time each day, and utilizing devices that make it easier to organize and remember. This includes traditional pill boxes and delivery systems as well as newer digital applications, such as Bluetooth reminders that will send reminders to take a medicine. There is also a feature of the Epilepsy Foundation's My Seizure Diary that allows careful tracking of medications and will send reminders (https://www .epilepsy.com/living-epilepsy/epilepsy-foundation-my-seizure-diary).

Blood Levels of Antiseizure Medications and the Therapeutic Range

One of the principal advances in our ability to control seizures came when we learned how to measure the amount (level) of an antiseizure medication in the blood and thus assess the amount of the medicine actually reaching the brain. Even now many physicians do not fully understand the use of blood levels and the concept of the *therapeutic range* of a given medication. Parents (and physicians) often believe that these levels ensure control of the seizures or guarantee the absence of side effects, misbeliefs that often lead to misuse of blood-level information. Also, some of the new medications act by mechanisms unrelated to the serum levels and therefore do not have established therapeutic ranges.

As mentioned above, blood levels are measured in the serum (liquid portion) of the blood, which may be taken by needle stick from a vein or by pricking the finger. (There are several different methods of measuring the drug level, but those techniques are not important here.) The test must be requested and interpreted by your child's physician and should always be done with proper quality control.

What is the correct blood level for your child? The correct blood level is the amount of the medication that controls the seizures. It is not a specific amount. The optimal level is the lowest level that works without causing toxicity. It will vary from one child to another.

The concept of the therapeutic range is often misunderstood. It may be useful to understand how the therapeutic ranges for these medications have been established. A small number of adults (or sometimes children) were carefully studied using a single medication. The lower end of the therapeutic range was then determined by the level at which seizures began to be controlled in a majority of these individuals. The upper end of the range was the point at which some individuals began to show signs of toxicity. Thus, the therapeutic range is the medication level at which most individuals are likely to have their seizures controlled without toxicity. Your child is not an average but an individual. Thus, they may require a higher-than-average level or a lower-than-average level to control the seizures. They may be able to tolerate more or less than average levels before showing signs of toxicity. Therefore, finding the correct dose of a given medicine for your child requires a trial to determine what is enough and what is too much for *your* child.

The therapeutic range is commonly believed to be the gold standard that will guarantee seizure control and avoid toxicity and side effects. It does neither. Yet many physicians misinterpret the therapeutic range as the range where they should keep the blood level, decreasing the dose of the medicine if the blood level is above the range and increasing it if the level is below the range.

To repeat, the correct blood level for your child is enough—*enough to control the seizures and not enough to cause toxicity. The therapeutic range is a guide, nothing more.*

Common Questions about Blood Levels

Physicians and parents have become enamored of tests and often give them greater importance than is proper. Despite scientific advances, the proper use of anticonvulsants remains an art, not a science. We are often asked such questions as these by both physicians and parents:

Q. *"My doctor says that my child's blood level is slightly low and wants to increase his dose. What should I do?"*

A. If you ask us this, we would ask if your child is still having seizures. If he is, then the dose should be increased. If he is not, then we would leave the dose alone; the current level appears to be sufficient to control his seizures. The question of increasing a dose often comes up in a child whose seizures are controlled. As the child grows and increases in size, the blood level will, of course, decrease if your doctor doesn't increase the dose. But we suggest keeping the dose the same as the child grows and gains weight, unless he begins to have seizures again. If the dose is kept the same, then the blood level gradually falls over the months or years. If the child does not have another seizure, it will be easier and safer to take him off his medicine when he has been free of seizures for two years. If he has a seizure, then you know that he needs to stay on the medication longer and that the dose may need to be increased.

Q. *"My daughter's blood level is at the upper end of 'normal,' and she is still having seizures. My doctor wants to try another drug. Is that the proper thing to do?"*
A. We would suggest first that your child's physician try increasing the dose even further, but slowly, since your daughter is close to the point where many people show toxicity. Sometimes seizures will be controlled with a little more medication without any toxic problems. The upper level of the therapeutic range is like a WARNING sign: it suggests that you and your child's physician should be watchful for signs of toxicity.

Q. *"Rachel's blood level is 'high,' and my doctor wants to lower the dose. I think that she is doing just fine, and she hasn't had any seizures since the last increase in dosage. What should we do?"*
A. We would recommend that you leave the dose alone. If Rachel isn't having any seizures and has no signs of toxicity, then perhaps this is the level she requires. Since the level is above the usual range, however, we would suggest that you keep a close eye on her and on her school performance, to be sure that the medication is not interfering, and that you stay alert for other signs of toxicity.

Q. *"Billy's blood level is right in the middle of the 'range.' Is that good?"*
A. The answer to this question is, "It depends." If Billy is not having any seizures and shows no signs of toxicity, then that level is fine and should not be changed. If he is still having seizures, then the level is too low for him, and he needs more medication. If he is too sleepy, too irritable, or having problems in school, then it is important to find out why. There are many causes for problems such as these. Obviously, you should be sure that he is not having seizures. If the level is not high, then the medication is a less likely cause of these problems. If you can't find another cause, however, then lowering or discontinuing the medicine may be worth trying. If the problem disappears, then it may have been due to the medication.

Q. *"How frequently must she have her blood levels of the anticonvulsant checked? She is really afraid of needles."*
A. If your child's seizures are not under control despite a good dose of medication, we may just increase the dose, or we may get a blood level to make certain that the child is taking the medicine, that they are absorbing it properly, and that they are not metabolizing it too fast. The blood levels do not tell you that they have enough, but they may guide your decisions when you want to give more or less. We do not do blood levels either frequently or routinely. Your child does not need a blood-level test every time they visit the doctor.

Choosing the Best Medication

All medications do not work equally well for every seizure type. Therefore it is necessary to classify the child's seizure. For each seizure type, there are several medications that are usually equally effective. The choice between them is then made on the basis of the medication's side effects, its cost, the child's age, and any previous drug allergies. Some medications are more effective for partial and tonic-clonic seizures, others for absence seizures. We discuss them in those groupings and in the order in which they were discovered.

Antiseizure Medications

The next sections discuss the more commonly used antiseizure medications (ASMs). Each medication is presented in a paragraph or two and focuses on the highlights of how and when we use it. For more information, especially on some of the newer medications, we encourage you to read about them on the internet, either at epilepsy.com or the pharmaceutical company's website. Of course, anything you read on the internet is subject to possible bias, so check with your child's neurologist if you have questions.

The Older Medications

This section focuses on some of the original, first generation of medications introduced to the market over the period 1910–93. This does not mean, in any way, that they are not helpful or useful just because they are not "modern." Several ASMs are still widely used, especially in pediatrics, namely ethosuximide (Zarontin) and valproate (Depakote). We have years of experience with these medications, and children do very well with them. The next section focuses on the second generation of ASMs, from 1994 to 2010, including commonly used medications like levetiracetam (Keppra), topiramate (Topamax), and lamotrigine (Lamictal) among others. Finally, we highlight the newest medications to become available in the United States in the last decade, including clobazam (Onfi) and cannabidiol (Epidiolex).

Phenobarbital (Luminal) is the second antiseizure medication ever discovered (bromides came first in 1853). Phenobarbital came onto the market in 1912 and has been used for more than one hundred years. It works on GABA receptors and is inhibitory (see Chapter 1). It comes in tablets, liquid (20 mg/5 ml), and intravenous preparations and is inexpensive. Phenobarbital today is mostly used for two reasons in children: (1) in infancy because of predictable absorption and levels, and a long history of use in the neonatal ICU; and (2) to help stop status epilepticus that does not respond to diazepam, lorazepam, levetiracetam, or phenytoin. Sometimes phenobarbital is tried when many of the newer medications are unsuccessful for a given child, as it can sometimes be helpful. It lasts a long time in the bloodstream and is often dosed once a day. Side effects are definitely a big issue and include sedation, effects on the liver, and sometimes negative effects on learning. It is a controlled substance.

Phenytoin (Dilantin) was discovered in 1936 and is one of the most widely used medications in the world for adults still today. Although it comes in a liquid formulation (125 mg/5 ml), the absorption of it in children is hard to predict, and levels can fluctuate significantly, even throughout the day—typically, it is dosed twice a day using tablets or capsules. It is usually helpful for focal seizures, not generalized ones. Phenytoin today, like phenobarbital, is mostly used in an emergency to stop active seizures, especially status epilepticus. When given for status epilepticus, it is typically given as a form of phenytoin called fosphenytoin, which is safer to give through an IV. Side effects include gum swelling, dizziness, coarse facial features (with long-term use), and decreased bone density.

Carbamazepine (Tegretol) is a medication that works on sodium channels and has been available since 1962. It is dosed twice a day, although it may work better if used three times a day. Carbamazepine is the gold-standard medication for focal epilepsy (and does not help, or can worsen, generalized epilepsy). It has largely been supplanted by modifications to the core molecule in medications such as oxcarbazepine (Trileptal) and eslicarbazepine (Aptiom), which were designed to have fewer side effects and are discussed in the next two sections. Carbamazepine comes in tablets, chewable tablets, and liquid formulations (100 mg/5 ml). Long-acting versions include Carbatrol and Tegretol XR. Side effects include changes in white blood cell counts, anemia, low platelets, liver function changes, dizziness, and rash. Over time, the carbamazepine levels can drift downward, which is called *autoinduction*. It means that the body metabolizes the medication more quickly. Serious skin rashes with carbamazepine are more common in Asians with the HLA-B1502 gene, which can be tested for (or this medication can be avoided in certain populations). Carbamazepine is also used for nerve pain and mood disorders.

Ethosuximide (Zarontin) has been used since 1960 and is one of the most popular first-line medications for absence seizures. A famous study published in 2010, comparing ethosuximide, valproate, and lamotrigine for absence seizures in children, found that it was equal in efficacy to valproate but had fewer side effects, making it the medication of first choice for this condition. Working on calcium channels, it does not help focal seizures. Ethosuximide comes in a liquid preparation (250 mg/5 ml) as well as gel capsules. Side effects include stomach upset (less common with the capsules and if taken with food, especially milk), blood count abnormalities (labs required), rash, and headache.

Valproate or valproic acid (Depakote or Depakene) was first available on the market in 1962 and has a broad spectrum of activity; in many ways it was the first *broad-spectrum* ASM for seizures, effective for many different seizure types. It is especially helpful for absence, myoclonic, tonic, and even focal seizures. Valproate is also useful for migraine and mood disorders. It is currently available in tablets, sprinkle capsules (which can be opened up into applesauce, yogurt, ice cream, etc.), liquid (250 mg/5 ml), and intravenously. Several extended-release tablets exist as well to allow it to be given once daily.

Unfortunately, the side effect profile can be intimidating, and as such, valproate is not as commonly used as years ago. Some new medications may be as effective. Valproate can cause weight gain. Because of increased appetite, but also for unclear reasons, children can gain weight even when eating their usual amounts. In addition, hair thinning, blood count abnormalities, liver changes, pancreatitis, ovarian cysts, polycystic ovary syndrome, and nausea can be seen. Perhaps the most worrisome side effect is teratogenicity; there is a much higher chance of a baby having birth defects or intellectual problems if the mother is taking valproate while pregnant. If valproate was taken and stopped years back, and the child is now an adult and pregnant, teratogenicity is not a problem. It is often avoided in adolescent girls to be on the safe side. Despite these problems, it is important to remember that valproate is one of the most effective antiseizure medications; it should be strongly considered (weighing the pros and cons) for any child with refractory epilepsy, or seizures that aren't controlled by other medications. In our experience, we occasionally see adolescent girls who have generalized epilepsy and have failed multiple ASMs, but no neurologist is willing to consider val-

proate. After proper consent about side effects and unplanned pregnan-
cies, these children have often done well with valproate.

Clonazepam (Klonopin), a benzodiazepine medication like diazepam (Valium) and clobazam (Onfi), first came on the market in 1975.
It comes in three strengths of tablets and five strengths of orally disinte-
grating wafers. Unlike diazepam, clobazam is more commonly used as a
daily ASM. Clonazepam, however, is more frequently used temporarily,
either due to a seizure cluster or as a bridge between one ASM and another if a change is being made. Similar to other benzodiazepines, it can
cause sedation, mood change, and dizziness. It also can lead to increased
drooling, which can be problematic for some people, especially those
with cerebral palsy.

Felbamate (Felbatol) was approved in 1993 by the FDA for the treatment of Lennox-Gastaut syndrome (see Chapter 8). Effectively targeting
GABA and NMDA receptors (Chapter 1), it has a unique and powerful
mechanism of action and can be helpful for difficult-to-control seizures.
It is available in tablets (400 and 600 mg) and liquid (600 mg/5 ml).

One year after its introduction, cases emerged of severe aplastic
anemia (loss of all blood cells from the bone marrow) and then liver
damage shortly afterward. Neurologists received a letter from the FDA
warning them of this and suggesting that it be used only in severe epilepsy where the benefits outweighed the risks. Today, it is used in children with Lennox-Gastaut syndrome where other medications have
failed, with blood counts and liver functions checked regularly. The risk
of aplastic anemia is low (1:5,000) and may be lower in children; liver
damage is uncommon as well (1:34,000). Our center has a few patients
on this medication, usually as they are doing well with it, but it is not
commonly used.

Gabapentin (Neurontin) is the final medication of this group of older
antiseizure medications. It was first approved in 1993 and works on calcium channels (despite its name sounding like it would affect GABA). It
is available in tablets, capsules, and a liquid formulation (250 mg/5 ml).
Gabapentin is known throughout the neurology community as helpful
for conditions other than epilepsy, including migraine, neuropathic pain
(especially due to diabetes), headache, sleep, and restless legs syndrome.

As an ASM, although it can help focal seizures, it is not commonly used because of relatively less efficacy than other medications. Side effects are few, however, and limited to mostly sleepiness and weight gain. We sometimes use gabapentin when there is combined epilepsy (focal and generalized) and pain or difficulty with sleep.

The following example shows how medications are changed in response to ongoing seizures to provide informed seizure control.

Samantha was an adolescent girl who developed absence epilepsy at age 9. Although she had a significant reduction in her absence seizures with ethosuximide, the seizures continued a few times per week. At age 12, she had a generalized tonic-clonic seizure, so her neurologist added lamotrigine. For the next few years, several newer medications were tried to control both her absence and generalized tonic-clonic seizures, but they continued, and she was becoming upset. At the age of 14, with her consent and after a long discussion about birth control, she was started on valproate. Within 2 weeks all her seizures stopped, and she has remained on valproate for the past 2 years, as well as oral contraceptives, and is now driving.

The Newer Medications

The antiseizure medications in this section are often referred to as third-generation medications. They have been developed in about the last 30 years. These medications have various mechanisms of action and often can be used in combination with each other or the medications in other sections if one medication alone is not controlling seizures. These medications sometimes have fewer side effects than the older medications, may require less blood work monitoring, and we have lots of experience with using them. We have some understanding of the long-term effects on health and safety in pregnancy. Of these medications Vimpat does not have a generic formulation at the time of this writing. These medications are typically covered easily by insurance, other than Vimpat, which often requires prior authorization.

Lamotrigine (Lamictal) is a sodium channel medication that works for both generalized and focal seizures. Another broad-spectrum medication, lamotrigine has few side effects and is tolerated well. It has the added benefit of sometimes helping mood. In some patients, including those with juvenile myoclonic epilepsy, it can sometimes increase myoclonic seizures, so be aware. There is a risk of serious rash with lamotrigine called Stevens-Johnson syndrome (SJS); however, SJS is quite rare if the medication is increased very slowly when starting it. For this reason, it takes up to 2 months to get a good starting dose. This medicine is safe in pregnancy, although its levels are affected by both birth control pills and pregnancy. Valproic acid also slows the metabolism of this medication, so if valproic acid is started while on lamotrigine, the lamotrigine dose often needs to be decreased. Blood levels are often followed on this medication. Lamotrigine levels are affected by pregnancy and need to be followed regularly with a neurologist during pregnancy.

Lamotrigine comes as dissolvable tablets (25, 50, 100, and 200 mg), chewable pills (2, 5, and 25 mg), and pills (25, 100, 150, and 200 mg). Side effects are few but include dizziness at high levels and risk of SJS.

Topiramate (Topamax) is a carbonic anhydrase inhibitor that works in various ways, including on sodium channels, GABA activity increasing inhibition, and glutamate receptors. All these factors lead to potentially decreasing the likelihood of seizure activity. Topiramate works for both generalized and focal seizures (broad spectrum). It is also used to treat headaches and tics in some people. Topamax comes as capsules with sprinkles inside (15 and 25 mg) and as tabs (25, 50, 100, and 200 mg). There is a long-acting form called Trokendi. This medication can be compounded into a liquid in some pharmacies. The most common side effects are decreased appetite and trouble thinking of the word you would like to say. Rare side effects include kidney stones and trouble sweating. It is a good idea to make sure your child is drinking plenty of water on this medication.

Zonisamide (Zonegran) works similarly to topiramate but also affects sodium and calcium channels. It can work well for both generalized and focal seizures, although it is often considered more of a first- or second-line medication for generalized seizures. It comes as capsules with powder inside (25, 50, and 100 mg) and can also be compounded into a liquid at some pharmacies. Zonisamide is a very long-acting medication, so it can typically be taken once a day. Some people find that at higher doses, taking it twice a day reduces side effects. Side effects are similar to topiramate but usually less common and less severe. So, if topiramate is not being well tolerated but seizures are controlled, zonisamide will likely be substituted.

Levetiracetam (Keppra) probably works through binding with the synaptic vesicle 2A (SV2A) receptor, but there may be other mechanisms not yet known. Levetiracetam works well for both generalized and focal seizures and is probably the most popular antiseizure drug in the United States currently. Levetiracetam is metabolized through the kidneys. The medication comes as both pills (250, 500, 750, and 1,000 mg) and liquid (100 mg/1 ml). Levetiracetam's main side effect is changes in mood. Some people will feel more irritable on the medicine, which typically manifests as having a short fuse, often noticed by family members and not the patients themselves. Levetiracetam has been shown to increase the risk of patients wanting to harm themselves (suicidal ideation). If there is a change in mood on the medication or sleepiness as a result of the medication, often adding a small dose (2 mg/kg up to a maximum dose of 100 mg per day) of vitamin B6 is helpful to counteract the side effects in about 30 percent. Be sure to ask your doctor the correct dose of B6 before starting it, as doses of B6 that are too high can cause peripheral neuropathy (tingling in the fingers and toes). Levetiracetam levels are affected by pregnancy and need to be followed regularly with a neurologist during pregnancy. Levetiracetam has been shown to be safe in pregnancy.

Vigabatrin (Sabril) works on GABA receptors. This medication is mostly used for infantile spasms in children (see Chapter 8), especially children with tuberous sclerosis complex, but it can also be used for focal epilepsy. It is obtained through a specialty pharmacy that delivers it directly to the patient. Side effects include permanent loss of peripheral vision, although this has not yet been shown to definitively occur when used for less than 6 months. It may also cause abnormalities on an MRI, which are called "unidentified bright objects," typically in the basal ganglia, and are of unclear significance but may cause temporary neurological complications depending on where they are located in the brain.

Lacosamide (Vimpat) works on sodium channels in a slightly different way than the other sodium channel medications. This is a good medicine for focal epilepsy and sometimes works for generalized epilepsy as well. There is no generic for this medication so it can sometimes take a little time to get it covered by insurance. It comes as pills (50, 100, 150, and 200 mg), intravenously, and also as a liquid (10 mg/1 ml). This medication does not require regular lab tests. Side effects are few and include dizziness at high doses.

Rufinamide (Banzel) has many mechanisms of action, including on the sodium channels. It is often used for generalized epilepsy, including atonic seizures, and in Lennox-Gastaut syndrome. It comes in tablets (200 and 400 mg) and as a liquid (40 mg/ml). This medicine affects the metabolism of other medicines, especially valproate, so levels often need to be monitored. Additionally, it can cause the white blood cell count to decrease, so labs are frequently obtained.

Oxcarbazepine (Trileptal) is a sodium channel medication that works well for focal epilepsy. It can rarely cause the sodium in the blood to decrease, and therefore blood work is often followed. Blood levels can also be helpful in adjusting the medication dosing. At high doses it can cause dizziness, especially in combination with outer sodium channel medications. Oxcarbazepine can decrease the effectiveness of hormonal birth control, so an alternate form of pregnancy protection should be used when on the medicine. Oxcarbazepine comes in liquid form (300 mg/5 ml) and in pill form (150, 300, and 600 mg). There is a long-acting form of oxcarbazepine called Oxtellar. This medication is related to carbamazepine and eslicarbazepine.

Jon-Michael began having seizures at the age of 5 and was diagnosed with childhood epilepsy with centrotemporal spikes after seeing a neurologist. His parents were very worried about antiseizure medications and knew that this type of epilepsy isn't always treated. After several bothersome seizures in the middle of the night, he was started on a low dose of levetiracetam, and seizures stopped completely. Levetiracetam was then stopped after 2 years and a normal EEG.

The Newest Medications

As of the writing of this book, in 2022, these antiseizure medications are the newest ones to come to market, but by no means are we saying that newest means the best. These medicines have had less time in use for us to really know their best uses and full range of side effects. For many of them, we have little experience in children and have to look at experience in adults and try to make them applicable to children. But children, as you know, aren't just small adults. In general, these newest medications are used after those in the previous two sections have been tried and were not efficacious. In some children, they are important for improved control. Nonetheless, because of less pediatric experience, significantly higher costs (and difficult insurance issues), and fewer trials in children, their use is somewhat limited.

Despite this, those of us in pediatric epilepsy are excited to see so many new options coming to local pharmacies for our patients. Most of these new medicines target mechanisms of action that are different from older medications, which means they might work differently (and maybe help a child who hasn't had success with drugs from the previous two sections). Of the eight medications in this section, only one (clobazam) currently has a generic option, but many have liquid preparations. They are not listed in any particular order. Importantly, cannabidiol (Epidiolex) is included in this chapter as it is a prescription antiseizure medication. Artisanal CBD (with or without THC) is discussed in more detail in Chapter 13, which deals with complementary and alternative treatments. These medications are new, and if strongly considering starting them for your child, beyond reading about them here, learn more at the Epilepsy Foundation website or ask your neurologist for resources to find out more—experience and information are growing rapidly.

Clobazam (Onfi) works on GABA receptors and is in the benzodiazepine family but is different from other benzodiazepines, like lorazepam and diazepam (Ativan and Valium); it is longer acting so that the body doesn't get used to it, and it can therefore be taken daily. In other words, it doesn't lose its effectiveness over time as would typically be seen with diazepam and lorazepam. Clobazam has been available for many years in Europe and Canada (under the name Frisium) and only recently came to the United States as an orphan drug with initial approval for Lennox-Gastaut syndrome in 2011. Studies in the United States, which led to its FDA approval, showed a dramatic improvement in the drop seizures (atonic) of Lennox-Gastaut syndrome, and we often use it today for this kind of seizure. Other good options for drop seizures include ketogenic diets and vagus nerve stimulation. Clobazam was initially very expensive (in the United States), and insurance companies made it difficult to prescribe unless the child specifically had Lennox-Gastaut syndrome. That has been slightly less of a logistical problem with the new generic version. Today it is one of the most popular of the antiseizure drugs for difficult-to-control pediatric epilepsy.

Clobazam comes in many preparations, including tablets (10 and 20 mg), liquid (2.5 mg/ml), and now a dissolvable strip that can be placed on a child's tongue called Sympazan, which comes in 5, 10, and 20 mg oral strips (that interestingly have nearly zero carbs for children on ketogenic diets). It is dosed typically twice a day. It is also sometimes helpful for anxiety. Clobazam works for both generalized and focal epilepsy. Side effects include sleepiness, mood changes, and sometimes increased appetite.

Perampanel (Fycompa) was approved in 2012 and works on AMPA receptors, which differs from other medications for seizures. It is approved by the FDA for adults and children over age 4 with focal epilepsy, but early experience suggests that it may be helpful for generalized epilepsy too. We have been using it for Lennox-Gastaut syndrome and other difficult-to-control seizure types. This medication (and the others to follow in this section) are available only by brand name (no generic) at this time, so be prepared for having to seek prior authorization from the insurance company and thus delays getting it.

Perampanel comes in tablets (2, 4, 6, 8, 10, and 12 mg) and a liquid (0.5 mg/ml) and is usually dosed once a day at night (but twice a day is okay too). We tend to use low doses in children, 2–4 mg/day. The main side effect that we've seen so far is mood change, specifically hostility, which is somewhat like levetiracetam and goes away when the medication is stopped or the dose is lowered. It can also cause dizziness.

Brivaracetam (Briviact) is a medication that works on the same receptor (SV2a) that levetiracetam targets. Brivaracetam is approved for focal epilepsy in adults and children over age 4. It comes in tablets (10, 25, 50, 75, and 100 mg), liquid (10 mg/ml), as well as an IV form. Since it works like levetiracetam, but maybe with fewer mood changes, it is usually used in those who did well with levetiracetam in terms of seizure control but had mood changes. Brivaracetam right now does not have much data in children, but that may change.

Eslicarbazepine (Aptiom) is the latest medication to modify and improve the molecule that is carbamazepine or the next generation oxcarbazepine. Eslicarbazepine is the S-isomer of oxcarbazepine (hence the *s* in the name). It is approved for focal seizures (and it does *not* help generalized seizures) in children over age 4. It currently comes in tablets (200, 400, 600, and 800 mg) and not liquid.

It is new and expensive, so usually insurance companies will suggest oxcarbazepine instead right now. We also do not have a lot of pediatric experience with Aptiom yet. It is used similarly to oxcarbazepine although can be given once a day at night and may have less chance of dizziness and double vision, but it has similar chance (about 4%) of hyponatremia (low sodium in the blood). Like oxcarbazepine, we suspect that when eslicarbazepine becomes a generic medication that it will be easier to prescribe, and it may supplant the previous oxcarbazepine medication in common use.

Stiripentol (Diacomit) is a new drug that is unique because it's an "aromatic alcohol." Like clobazam, it has been widely used in Europe since 2001; it came to the United States in 2018. It is specifically approved for the treatment of children aged 2 or older with Dravet syndrome (see Chapter 8). In addition, the child must also be on valproate and sometimes clobazam as well depending on insurance companies.

It comes in capsules (250 and 500 mg) and a powder (250 and 500 mg) that can be added to water and turned into a liquid. At this time, it is prescribable only through an independent specialty pharmacy. The mechanism of action is not clear but appears to be through GABA. Stiripentol is dosed twice a day, and it is recommended that physicians check blood counts periodically for low white blood cells. It interacts with other drugs, so be careful, as it can raise their levels (especially clobazam, which may be a good thing—see cannabidiol later in this section). Other side effects include loss of appetite and drowsiness.

Fenfluramine (Fintepla) has been approved for the treatment of Dravet syndrome in children over age 2 years (June 2020). Similar to stiripentol and cannabidiol, it has this specific indication. It is very expensive and typically requires having Dravet syndrome to be approved by insurance companies. It works on serotonin receptors, which is new for an antiseizure drug, and comes in a liquid preparation (2.2 mg/ml). Originally *fen-phen* (fenfluramine combined with another drug, phentermine) was a weight-loss drug that was pulled from the US market because of thickening of the heart valves. In clinical trials in children at a much lower dose (just the fenfluramine component), this was not seen, but the FDA has required echocardiograms (ultrasounds of the heart) to be done before starting and then every 6 months in children receiving this drug, including after it has been stopped. It also has to be obtained from a specialty pharmacy.

Cannabidiol (Epidiolex) was approved in 2018 in the United States (2019 in Europe as Epidyolex) as the first (probably of many) prescribable pharmaceutical-grade cannabidiol (CBD). Unlike artisanal products, this is nearly 100 percent CBD. In other words, the antiseizure medication (CBD) has been purified from cannabis (marijuana) and the more psychoactive THC. It was originally a Schedule V substance (meaning one-month only, special prescriptions), but that is no longer the case as the FDA realized there is no chance of abuse. Cannabidiol targets cannabinoid receptors, which is unique. Similar to many other medications in this section, it is approved for children aged 1 year and over with either Dravet syndrome or Lennox-Gastaut syndrome. It has most recently been approved for use in tuberous sclerosis complex as well. Because of the very high cost ($30,000/year), it is scrutinized by insurance companies, including for refills. It currently comes in a liquid formulation (100 mg/ml) that arrives by FedEx and has a strawberry flavor; dosing is twice a day. It is mixed in sesame oil, and levels can be higher with high fat meals (so be careful on ketogenic diets).

Just like artisanal CBD products (see Chapter 13), it is a medical option with real side effects. Liver function tests can be significantly elevated (especially if the child is also taking valproate) and should be checked regularly. Children can become sleepy and have decreased appetite. Clobazam levels can increase up to three times when cannabidiol is started, so often clobazam levels need to be checked or the dose lowered. In our experience this is a helpful medication, especially for Dravet syndrome, and parents often want it refilled after a one-month trial.

Cenobamate (Xcopri) is the newest antiseizure medication at the writing of this book, having been FDA approved and available since May 2020. It works uniquely through sodium channels and GABA. It is currently approved for adults 18 and older with focal epilepsy, so any pediatric use is new and may not be approved by insurance companies easily.

Cenobamate impressed many neurologists with a very high (28%) seizure-free rate in clinical trials of very medication-refractory patients, so there is some excitement about this new medication. Main side effects include sedation and dizziness, but a rare condition called DRESS (drug reaction with eosinophilia and systemic symptoms), basically a very severe rash with blood and liver abnormalities, happened in three people in the trials. DRESS seems to be much less common if the doses are increased very slowly, hence the availability of a starter pack and many strengths of tablets (12.5, 25, 50, 100, 150, and 200 mg). It may interact with phenytoin and clobazam, along with lamotrigine. For more information on cenobamate, we would suggest epilepsy.com or sites recommended by your neurologist.

Brittany had epilepsy due to Lennox-Gastaut syndrome and had tried and failed ten antiseizure drugs and the ketogenic diet. She was on valproate, topiramate, and clobazam but continued to have daily seizures. Her father was worried that no medications would ever control her seizures. Cannabidiol was started, and her seizures improved, but she became very sleepy. Her neurologist lowered the clobazam dose by 30 percent and she became more awake. Now 6 months later, she is not seizure-free, but she is having fewer larger seizures and visits to the emergency department.

CHAPTER 11

Rescue Medicine and Treatment of Status Epilepticus

When your child has a seizure or is diagnosed with epilepsy, your child's doctor may discuss providing you with a rescue medication. A rescue medication is a medicine that is given to stop a seizure while someone is seizing or to stop a cluster of seizures (multiple seizures in a row). Typically, it is recommended that if a child seizes for longer than 5 minutes, a rescue medication be administered. This is because it can become harder to stop a seizure once it has been going on for this long. The recommended time to give a rescue medication may vary somewhat from patient to patient, however. This is particularly true if you live a long way from care or if your child typically has prolonged seizures. Your doctor may prescribe a rescue medicine to give if your child has a seizure that is longer than usual.

Status Epilepticus

The classic definition of status epilepticus is a seizure that lasts longer than 30 minutes, but we now typically define status epilepticus as a seizure that lasts longer than 5 minutes because after 5 minutes, experience has shown that a seizure is often harder to stop. It is also considered status epilepticus if someone has multiple seizures in a row without coming back to their normal function in between.

There are many possible causes of status epilepticus. It can be a consequence of infection of the brain, such as meningitis or encephalitis. It can be due to head trauma, brain tumors, or other serious causes.

Sometimes the reason is unknown. Children with epilepsy can also develop status epilepticus. Whatever the cause, it is important to stop the seizures as quickly as possible.

There are two types of status epilepticus. The more common type is convulsive status epilepticus, where you can see the seizures. The other type is nonconvulsive status epilepticus, which does not involve any movements that you can see. This type is rare. One type of epilepsy where nonconvulsive status epilepticus appears, although rarely, is in absence seizures. If this occurs, a child may appear confused, wandering, not answering questions appropriately, or acting much slower or duller than usual. A change such as this could also be due to medication or illness, so if you see these symptoms, you should contact your child's doctor. They may recommend an EEG to better diagnose the problem.

Rescue medications can be used at home and at the hospital to treat status epilepticus. If using medications at home and the seizure does not stop within a few minutes of giving the medicine, then emergency help should be called. These rescue medications are different forms of the class of medication called benzodiazepines. Most benzodiazepines are fast acting and can therefore be used to stop a seizure when it is occurring. There are different types of rapidly acting benzodiazepines, and there are different ways to give them. It's also important to remember to continue giving your child their routine medications. The fast-acting benzodiazepines are meant only for short-term relief. It's important to give the full dose that is prescribed by your doctor.

Diazepam (Valium, Diastat) is a benzodiazepine that can be given in various ways. It is most commonly prescribed as a rectal gel (Diastat). This can be injected (like giving an enema) into the rectum for prolonged seizures using a premade cardboard applicator with jelly. Diazepam is also available as a very concentrated liquid (Intensol), which can be placed between the teeth and gums, where it is absorbed, during a seizure. Normally we tell people not to put something into a person's mouth when they're having a seizure, but your child doesn't need to be able to swallow for the medication to work. They won't choke on it. A nasal spray containing diazepam called Valtoco is also available. This nasal spray can be used for children as well and comes in 5 mg and

10 mg doses. It is currently recommended for use in stopping seizure clusters.

Lorazepam (Ativan) can also be obtained as a liquid, which can be absorbed between the teeth and gums during an ongoing seizure, or as a pill to help with seizure clusters. The liquid formulation, known as an Ativan Intensol preparation, needs to be refrigerated. This makes it difficult to carry with you on an emergency basis, although some families carry it in a cooler pack. Lorazepam is often what is given via IV or as an injection if someone presents to the hospital with ongoing seizures. This medication is also sometimes prescribed for use on a tapering schedule. If someone is having more frequent seizures than usual, possibly because of illness or other cause, lorazepam may be prescribed in progressively decreasing doses over several days to help calm the increase in seizures. It can also be used during transitions between medications.

Midazolam is most commonly used intranasally but can be used as an injection or given through the IV by emergency medical services or in the hospital. The newest formulation is prescribed as a nasal spray. Nayzilam is available only in adult doses (5 mg) and is FDA approved for children over age 12 years, at the time of this writing, so it is difficult to use in young children. Some pharmacies can dispense midazolam in a premeasured syringe attached to an atomizer, however, which can be used at lower doses. Midazolam in the injectable form is one of the most common medications that you will find in an ambulance.

Clonazepam is slightly longer acting than the other benzodiazepines that we've mentioned. This means that it also takes slightly longer to start working. It is most effective in stopping a cluster of seizures but can also be used to stop a single seizure. This medication is available as a dissolvable wafer for ease of administration and as a pill.

Another important benzodiazepine, clobazam (Onfi), is a very long-acting benzodiazepine and therefore cannot be used for rescue to stop an ongoing seizure. Enough of it won't get into your child's system to be of help on an emergency basis.

All the short-acting benzodiazepines have the side effect of making people sleepy. Some children have the opposite reaction when taking these medications, however, and will become agitated for a time.

If you use a rescue medication at home and it is not effective in stopping a seizure, then call 911. The most common medication that EMS will use to treat ongoing seizures is midazolam, which can be given as an injection.

If the use of benzodiazepines does not stop a seizure, then other medications will be used via IV at the hospital to try to do so. The most likely medications to be used next at the hospital to stop a seizure include fosphenytoin/phenytoin (Dilantin), levetiracetam (Keppra), or valproic acid (Depakote). These will be given as an intravenous load, which is a large dose of the medicine given through the IV. Should seizures continue, intravenous drip medications may be needed, and a child is admitted to the intensive care unit (ICU) when these are given so that they can be closely monitored. This is important to do because these other, more powerful medications can sometimes suppress breathing and other vital body functions.

CHAPTER 12

Ketogenic Diet Therapy

Ketogenic diet therapy has been a scientifically proven, nonpharmacologic treatment for epilepsy since 1921, more than one hundred years ago. It was first created at the Mayo Clinic in Rochester, Minnesota, as a sustainable way to mimic fasting and starvation diets, which had been used for several decades by faith healers. Although we know now that fasting and the ketogenic diet are completely separate treatments (and both work), these two treatments have been linked ever since.

For the next 20 years, the classic ketogenic diet was popular, as there were few other antiseizure medications available, and research flourished at the Mayo Clinic, Harvard, and Johns Hopkins. In the 1940s and especially 1950s, articles about the ketogenic diet dwindled, possibly as the new generation of neurologists didn't believe people would follow such a rigid diet and researchers interested in the diet moved on to other fields. In the 1960s and 1970s, new antiseizure drugs emerged on the scene, and the ketogenic diet was perceived as unnecessary, antiquated, and to be used only as a last resort in children with refractory epilepsy. Things changed dramatically in 1994 with the creation of the Charlie Foundation, which was named after a young boy named Charlie Abrahams who became seizure-free after starting the ketogenic diet here at Johns Hopkins under the guidance of Dr. John Freeman and his dietitian, Millicent Kelly. The ketogenic diet has since been studied and used further and is one of the mainstream treatments alongside drugs, surgery, and neurostimulation today.

We are now in a renaissance of sorts for dietary therapy as we approach its second century. Five different forms of diets can be used to treat seizures. The ways in which we start the diet, long based in tradition, have been challenged in meaningful and creative studies. Side effects have been well described and are often prevented by various supplements. New indications, including for conditions outside childhood epilepsy, have emerged on the scene. Biannual conferences with 500-plus attendees have been held all over the world for ketogenic diet practitioners; several published guidelines and consensus statements exist to guide expert management; and a new society, INKS (International Neurological Ketogenic Society), has been created (www.neuroketo.org).

This chapter provides some basic information about diet therapy for interested parents and children. In addition, the Johns Hopkins ketogenic diet team has recently published the updated seventh edition of their book *Ketogenic Diet Therapies for Epilepsy and Other Conditions*. We encourage you to read this book if after this chapter you want to learn more information. There is also additional ketogenic diet news at *Keto News* (www.epilepsy.com/ketonews), a blog on the latest science and happenings. When used for epilepsy, especially in children, however, we do not recommend starting the ketogenic diet on your own without medical guidance.

What Is the Ketogenic Diet?

The classic ketogenic diet is a high fat, moderate protein, low carbohydrate diet in which foods are carefully weighed and measured using a gram scale to create a particular ratio of grams of fat to protein and carbohydrate combined. A typical ratio is either 3:1 or 4:1, meaning that the ratio of grams of fat to grams of protein and carbohydrate together is 3:1 or 4:1. That means that 80–90 percent of the calories a child consumes are in the form of fats. Neurologists and dietitians work together to calculate an individual ratio and calories for a child. This (and other ketogenic diets) create a state of ketosis, in which the body breaks down fats instead of carbohydrates for energy. Ketone bodies can be measured in urine, blood, and breath, and they indicate that the body has made the metabolic shift but are not necessarily why the diet works. The mechanism of action of the diet is still not fully understood, but there are many possibilities. Several things happen to metabolism in the liver and brain when someone is on a ketogenic diet. Fatty acids are broken down in the liver into ketone bodies. These ketone bodies cross back into the blood, then go into the brain and are used by the TCA cycle to make energy (ATP) to fuel brain functions. If you do not provide glucose to the brain and instead give ketones, the brain does a nice job using those ketones to create energy.

The diet is traditionally started in the hospital over 2–3 days, including a brief 1-day fasting period (water and sugar-free liquids allowed). Many centers now do not have patients fast at the onset of the diet, and some even have people start the diet as outpatients. The recent COVID-19 pandemic has also led to creative ways to start the diet, including by telemedicine. The classic ketogenic diet is the most studied diet but also the strictest.

There are four other variations on the diet that are also available:

1. The medium chain triglyceride (MCT) diet was created in 1970 and uses MCT fats (e.g., coconut oil) in preference to other sources of fats/lipids to induce high levels of ketosis. MCTs are more ketogenic, which then allows for more carbohydrates in the meal plan. MCT fats can lead to gastrointestinal upset, however, and the percentage of MCT is carefully adjusted upward to avoid this. This diet is used widely in the UK and Canada.

2. The modified Atkins diet (MAD) was created in 2001 at Johns Hopkins based initially on parents reporting that their children could achieve ketosis and seizure control without sticking to a tight ratio or calorie count. This encourages considerably more protein to be incorporated into the diet while still restricting carbohydrates. Since then, now more than 20 years later, we have used this preferentially for adolescents and also adults on diet therapy. It is started at home after an in-person teaching session, and parents restrict carbohydrates to no more than 20 grams per day while encouraging fats and fluids. This diet is flexible and has advantages in being less strict than the classic ketogenic or MCT diets, but it also typically has less guidance from dietitians and the ability to be fine-tuned.

3. The low glycemic index treatment (LGIT) was created in 2005 at Massachusetts General Hospital based on the historical observation that some children on ketogenic diets lose seizure control with small carbohydrate indiscretions, even while maintaining ketosis. The LGIT diet is similar in many ways to the MAD, but the focus is on the glycemic index of carbohydrates. This involves using carbohydrates that cause the body to produce less insulin to metabolize them and allows much more freedom in choosing carbohydrates with a glycemic index of <55. Tables exist to find this glycemic index.

4. Finally, the modified ketogenic diet (MKD) was created several years ago in the UK as a way to allow the additional protein of the MAD but still maintain more strict control as in the classic ketogenic diet. A ratio of approximately 1:1 is targeted (75% fat, 20% protein, 5% carbohydrates), and household measures can also be used (rather than a gram scale). Publications on this diet are limited at this time.

All five diets are generally similar, with high fat and low carbohydrate foods. These foods may include bacon, eggs, mayonnaise, oils, heavy whipping cream, avocado, nuts, tuna fish, hamburger, and some carefully selected vegetables. There are also store-bought packaged low carb foods that may be acceptable on the ketogenic diet. Additionally, there are several prepared ketogenic diet formulas for use in infants and children with feeding tubes, including KetoCal and KetoVie. All five of these diets also seem to work similarly in terms of seizure control. Your child's neurologist and dietitian should be able to discuss the pros and cons of each therapy and help you decide what might be best for your child and your family.

How Well Does It Work?

Many studies, including randomized and controlled trials, show similar results. In children with difficult-to-control seizures, after 6 months, about 50–60 percent will be *responders*, meaning at least a 50 percent reduction in seizure frequency. About 10–15 percent of children starting the ketogenic diet will become seizure-free. This appears to be true independent of age, gender, region of the world, and how the diet is started. There are definitely some children, though, who do better than this with dietary therapy.

The diet can work quickly, sometimes within days, but usually we give it 2–3 months to reduce seizures before giving up. If effective, we traditionally keep children on the diet for 2 years, although some studies have suggested shorter periods may be equally appropriate. Just like antiseizure medications, we try to wean most children off ketogenic diets after a period to see if seizure control is maintained without it. Also, like ASMs, we usually wean the diet over time and do not abruptly discontinue it.

Who Does It Work Best For?

Over the years, it has become clear that diet therapy works extremely well for some conditions (*indications*), with better results than described previously. These indications are those in which more than 70 percent of children respond, or in the particular case of Glut1 deficiency (a condition often associated with epilepsy in which children cannot get glucose, the brain's fuel, across their blood-brain-barrier), a 95 percent responder rate. These conditions are listed below in alphabetical order, as published in the 2018 international ketogenic diet consensus guideline. There is more information about several of these conditions throughout this book. These are by no means the only conditions that diets can help. Every child, with rare exceptions, can theoretically be started on diet therapy to see if it helps. Ask your child's neurologist.

Indications

Angelman syndrome

Complex 1 mitochondrial disorders

Dravet syndrome

Epilepsy with myoclonic-atonic seizures (Doose syndrome)

Febrile infection-related epilepsy syndrome (FIRES)

Formula-fed-only infants or children

Glucose transporter protein 1 (Glut1) deficiency syndrome

Infantile spasms

Ohtahara syndrome

Pyruvate dehydrogenase deficiency

Super-refractory status epilepticus

Tuberous sclerosis complex

Katherine was an 18-month-old girl who had infantile spasms due to tuberous sclerosis complex. Vigabatrin had slowed down her spasms but not stopped them. She was completely formula fed because of difficulty swallowing foods. Her parents wanted to try the ketogenic diet, and her neurologist agreed. She stopped having spasms after 6 months and was able to stop two of her three antiseizure drugs too. After 2 years, the diet was slowly stopped, and she has done well, with very rare seizures and only a single antiseizure drug. Her parents still keep her sugar intake low, but she is otherwise back on regular formula and now foods.

What Are the Side Effects?

Ketogenic diet therapies are similar to all other therapies in this part of the book—they work, and they also have potential side effects. The good news is that most side effects are preventable, unlike some due to antiseizure drugs. Also, if a side effect does happen, usually we don't need to stop the ketogenic diet to make it go away.

The more common side effects are gastrointestinal: constipation, hunger, nausea, vomiting, weight loss. Occasional adverse effects include a ketosis that is too deep, growth slowing, high cholesterol levels, kidney stones, and bone density changes. More rare side effects are vitamin deficiency, pancreatitis, carnitine deficiency, and prolonged QT intervals. Today we prevent many of these side effects with supplements, such as a good multivitamin, calcium, vitamin D, carnitine, selenium, citrates, and several others. During a ketogenic diet admission, we spend a lot of time discussing with parents side effects to watch out for.

What Is in the Future of the Ketogenic Diet?

It is a very exciting time as many doctors are interested in diet therapy. Already today we're seeing increased use for infants, adolescents, and adults. In the next several years, we will likely see continued studies looking at the ketogenic diet as a first-line therapy, instead of waiting until many drugs have failed. It is also being used in very difficult-to-control status epilepticus. Trials looking at the diet for Alzheimer disease, migraines, autism, brain cancer, and other conditions beyond epilepsy will continue.

CHAPTER 13

Alternative and Complementary Therapies for Epilepsy

In this chapter we discuss some other options outside traditional medicine for the treatment of epilepsy. By definition, *alternative* means they are used instead of standard treatments (e.g., diet, medication, neurostimulation, and surgery), whereas *complementary* means they are used together with them. Most of these treatments unfortunately have little scientific evidence in the form of clinical trials (or FDA guidance) to support their use. That does not mean, however, that there is no experience in or value to using them. This chapter also includes artisanal CBD/THC (a nonpharmaceutical product produced with varying amounts of cannabidiol and tetrahydrocannabinol, which can produce sedation), along with steroids and intravenous immunoglobulin (IVIG), which one could argue are technically drugs that could be prescribed. There are many alternative/complementary therapies that we will not discuss in detail because there is really no scientific evidence of their efficacy, although we know that many families may explore their use. These include acupuncture, massage therapy, chiropractic manipulations, craniosacral-massage therapy, homeopathy, and hyperbaric oxygen and carbon dioxide therapy.

We encourage you to read in detail about any of these treatments you plan to try and ask other parents who have tried them for advice. Even if your neurologist is not familiar or supportive of you using an alternative or complementary therapy, it is *critical* that you mention it during a clinic visit, as sometimes these therapies interact with traditional treatments or increase the risk of seizures. An integrative physician who uses these treatments may also be willing to correspond and work with your neurologist.

Vitamins
With the exception of pyridoxine-dependency seizures, epilepsy is not typically due to a vitamin deficiency. In addition, megadoses of vitamins can have side effects. Despite this, some vitamins have been reported to be helpful complementary treatments for patients with epilepsy. These include pyridoxine (B6), which may also help the moodiness that can arise from taking levetiracetam, thiamine (B1), magnesium, vitamin E, and omega 3 fatty acids. Calcium with vitamin D, along with a standard multivitamin (e.g., Flintstones), is a reasonable addition to an antiseizure drug in many children because of concerns of the effect of certain ASMs on bone health.

Acupuncture
Acupuncture uses small needles to ease chronic pain based on traditional Chinese medicine. There are mixed results for migraine and pain, but it is widely used as a complementary therapy in many holistic practices. At this time, there is no evidence of its efficacy in epilepsy.

Artisanal CBD/THC (Medical Marijuana)
This alternative therapy is popular today because of the significant interest in medical marijuana in recent years, largely due to the benefits seen in a young girl named Charlotte Figi from Colorado. A special entitled "Weed" on CNN with Dr. Sanjay Gupta raised awareness about the possible role of medical marijuana in childhood epilepsy in 2013. Charlotte unfortunately passed away due to seizures from her underlying Dravet syndrome. Although medical marijuana has been used for epilepsy for perhaps five thousand years, this CNN special stimulated public awareness and led to research, including the introduction of the antiseizure drug cannabidiol (CBD, Epidiolex; see Chapter 10).

The research behind the use of artisanal CBD products, where the amounts of CBD and THC (tetrahydrocannabinol) may vary greatly and are usually obtained from state-licensed dispensaries, has shown benefits in the range of 25 percent of children with >50 percent seizure reduction, which is less than most ASMs. Studies have also shown adverse effects just like the ASM cannabidiol, including elevated clobazam levels and liver function changes. Artisanal CBD is certainly cheaper than cannabidiol overall, but it does cost approximately $200 a month and is not covered by insurance. To obtain artisanal CBD, families typically need to see a specified local provider to get a license to purchase medical marijuana. At this time, there is no scientific evidence that THC is helpful for epilepsy, and in our experience, some children can have increased seizures from it.

These products are not FDA regulated, so it is important to ask the dispensary exactly what is in them and get their advice on appropriate dosing. Store- or internet-purchased products can be obtained without a prescription, including from vendors like Charlotte's Web and Haleigh's Hope. Many hospitals do not allow unprescribed forms of CBD into the building due to the presence of small amounts of THC in the product. Additionally, most neurologists are not legally allowed by their hospital to provide medical advice about these substances.

At this time, we have less robust scientific evidence regarding these forms of CBD than the antiseizure drug cannabidiol. If insurance will not cover cannabidiol by prescription, however, the family often obtains artisanal CBD from a licensed dispensary or company and is guided with good advice about dosing. Its use is certainly reasonable if other antiseizure drugs have been tried and failed.

Just as with any therapy in this chapter, it is important to tell your child's neurologist if you have obtained and plan to start artisanal CBD. At our center, even though we cannot give medical advice about dosing, we do check liver function tests and may lower the clobazam dose (if the child is on that as well) to provide the best, safest care. More information is available at "Treating Seizures and Epilepsy," Epilepsy Foundation, https://www.epilepsy.com/learn/treating-seizures-and-epilepsy /other-treatment- approaches/medical-marijuana-and-epilepsy.

Herbs

Herbs are available at many local health-food stores and have increased in popularity in recent years for many medical conditions. In the treatment of epilepsy, several have been reported as helpful and appear on many websites. These include mugwort, valerian, burning bush, mistletoe, lily of the valley, and skullcap. These herbs are not FDA regulated and may have side effects; make sure you follow the instructions of an integrative physician, especially if used in children. Some Chinese (specifically from a moss plant), Japanese, and Indian herbs are under investigation as well for benefit in epilepsy. There are also some herbs to probably avoid, including gingko, garlic, and St. John's wort, which may affect the blood levels of antiseizure medications or lower the seizure threshold. For more information, see the informative article "About Herbs, Botanicals, and Other Products" on Memorial Sloan Kettering Cancer Center's website: https://www.mskcc.org/cancer-care/diagnosis-treatment/symptom-management/integrative-medicine/herbs.

Melatonin

The natural hormone melatonin is made by the pineal gland of the brain and can be purchased widely for helping children and adults to fall asleep, but it doesn't sustain sleep. Studies for its use for epilepsy have been mixed—some have shown benefit, while others have not. At this time, we tend to use it mostly as a sleep aid in those with epilepsy and insomnia, and if sleep abnormalities can be improved, then sometimes seizures improve as well.

Biofeedback

Biofeedback is a method of using imagery or relaxation to then influence body factors such as heart rate, breathing, or seizures. There is established evidence of its efficacy for pain and migraine. Some biofeedback centers will use an EEG along with biofeedback and try to change the rhythms of the brain. Studies have not shown benefit for epilepsy control, but the downside to trying these techniques is minimal, other than cost and time.

Yoga and Stress Relief

Relaxation techniques are being increasingly recognized as potentially helpful to reduce stress, which can be a trigger for epilepsy. Some recent publications in epilepsy journals have shown that reducing stress can also help seizures. There are various techniques, phone apps, and websites that can help parents and children learn ways to do reduce stress at home. For more information, go to the Epilepsy Foundation's Wellness Institute at https://www.epilepsy.com/living-epilepsy/healthy-living /stress-and-wellness.

Steroids

There is a limited role for corticosteroids (e.g., prednisolone, ACTH) in the treatment of epilepsy, but with very rare exception, the cause for seizures is *not* usually inflammation. These are drugs and not necessarily "alternative," but their standard use for epilepsy is not well established in most circumstances, so we discuss them in this chapter. The most established reasons to use steroids are infantile spasms, Landau-Kleffner syndrome, electrical status epilepticus of sleep, and refractory status epilepticus. In these forms of epilepsy, high dose steroids are used, recognizing that the high rate of side effects (e.g., weight gain, high blood pressure, increased infection rate, gastrointestinal upset) are sometimes appropriate given the benefits. Steroids are also sometimes used for epilepsy with myoclonic-atonic seizures (Doose syndrome), although the ketogenic diet is more effective, and sometimes steroids can aggravate the larger convulsions in this syndrome.

Intravenous Immunoglobulin

Intravenous immunoglobulin (IVIG) is a purified blood product obtained from donors and then given to a patient as an IV infusion over several hours to potentially bind antigens in their blood. It has well-established uses for some conditions, such as Guillain-Barré syndrome, but its use for epilepsy is not generally justified. One study with a placebo arm found no benefit to IVIG, and most recent reviews do not support its use. It is used for Landau-Kleffner syndrome, Rasmussen's syndrome, Lennox-Gastaut syndrome, and infantile spasms on rare occasions.

Jeremy's parents wanted to try a more "natural" approach to treat his seizures than standard antiseizure medications. He had tried levetiracetam and become very moody, so they had stopped it several months prior. They asked his neurologist for other options, and she recommended trying another medication, but they were insistent. Although their neurologist couldn't prescribe CBD/THC products, she supported their decision and noted it in her medical record. Jeremy's parents purchased it over the internet and came up with a dose based on what other parents and the company had suggested. He didn't have a seizure for a few months but then started having them again, and changing the amount of CBD/THC didn't help. After some discussion, they agreed to stop CBD/THC and start oxcarbazepine. He stopped having seizures completely and this time without any side effects. Neither his parents nor his neurologist was upset that they had tried alternative options and were glad they kept each other informed.

CHAPTER 14

Surgery and Devices

Antiseizure medications are the first line in treating epilepsy. Unfortunately, even with the development of many new medications, there are still about one-third of patients who will not be completely seizure-free on medicine. When medication does not control seizures, then other treatment options are considered. These include dietary therapy such as the ketogenic diet (Chapter 12) and surgical options.

There are two types of surgery we consider. These include resective surgery, where we remove the seizure focus (the area where the seizures start), and device placement.

When someone has failed two seizure medicines that were increased to high doses (not just failing a medication due to side effects) without controlling seizures, then their epilepsy is considered to be intractable, or refractory to medication. When that happens, we consider whether we can identify an area of the brain where the seizures are starting, and if so, whether removal of this area would improve, or ideally eliminate, seizures without creating a significant deficit for the patient.

When should we think about surgery? Surgery should not be the last alternative; it should be among the first things thought about. Thinking about surgery for epilepsy is not the same as doing epilepsy surgery. Research shows that once seizures have become intractable to medication (failed two medicines), the likelihood of another antiseizure medicine working is very low, and it is time to consider other seizure treatment options.

• *If* the seizures come from one area and that area can be easily removed without causing problems, surgery should be done, and earlier rather than later.

• *If* the epilepsy is caused by a lesion, a developmental problem of the brain, a cyst, or a tumor, then the seizures may be less likely to respond to medication. You and your child's physician should know whether surgery is or is not an option early in the course and at least think about surgery as an alternative.

Contemplating surgery is overwhelming. Except in the rare instance of a rapidly growing brain tumor, this surgery is not an emergency. Epilepsy surgery should never be placed "on the fast track." It should be done only after careful consideration of its potential risks and benefits.

The first clue that a patient might be helped by surgery is the nature of the seizures themselves. Are they focal in nature? Can we point to an area of the brain that we think the seizure may be coming from? Another early hint that the seizure might be focal is evidence from the routine EEG. To determine the location of the seizure focus, we always obtain imaging of the brain. Typically, we start with an MRI, which can look for changes in the way the brain formed or structural lesions that can be causing the brain to be irritable and therefore lead to seizures. Sometimes additional imaging is needed, and we may use imaging such as a position emission tomography (PET) scan, which looks for sugar (radioactive glucose) uptake in the brain (with lower sugar uptake than expected, indicating an area of the brain that may not be working as well); magnetoencephalography (MEG), which uses strong magnets to look for a seizure focus; or a SPECT scan (a nuclear medicine study that looks for how a seizure spreads).

In addition to imaging, the child will often be referred for long-term EEG monitoring, called *phase I monitoring.* The child will be admitted to the hospital and monitored on EEG, with a video recording, for a number of days to capture multiple seizures and determine where they are starting. Medications will often be weaned during this hospital stay so that the doctors are able to see more seizures.

Neuropsychological testing is also helpful in determining the seizure focus, as well as whether there are risks to taking out certain parts of the brain. This type of testing is much more extensive than routine psychological or psychoeducational testing that may be needed for educational evaluations. Neuropsychological evaluation is focused on brain-behavior relationships, and it measures an individual's cognitive strengths and weaknesses as they relate to specific brain functioning. This evaluation examines specific functions that might have been compromised because the seizures are coming from that particular part of the brain (or because of medications, or frequent seizures). In addition, neuropsychological evaluation can assist with identifying the cognitive risks of surgery. For instance, if a child has seizures that seem to be coming from the left temporal lobe, it would not be surprising to see that their language abilities and verbal memory are adversely affected. This functionality is examined even more closely if the child moves on to intracranial monitoring (phase II).

After phase I evaluation, imaging, and neuropsychological testing are completed, your child's team will discuss the next best steps in terms of considering surgery.

In some cases, phase II monitoring is recommended, which involves a surgery to place electrodes in or on the brain to get an even more precise understanding of where the seizures are coming from (see examples of surface and depth electrodes in Figure 14.1). In addition, this form of monitoring can inform us of the function of that particular area of the brain in order to determine if there is an area that is safe to remove. We are able to stimulate small parts of the brain to transiently stop those small areas from working. This doesn't hurt because the brain does not have pain sensors. In doing this we can see how losing function of a small area, for a moment, affects function. If function is affected, this gives us an idea whether there will be any loss of function when that area of the brain is surgically removed or ablated with laser surgery.

Phase II monitoring may consist of placing electrodes on the brain or deep in the brain. To place electrodes on the brain, the neurosurgeon will either create a small whole in the skull or remove a piece of the skull (craniotomy), place the electrodes, and then replace the skull so that seizures can then be monitored while your child is awake in the epilepsy

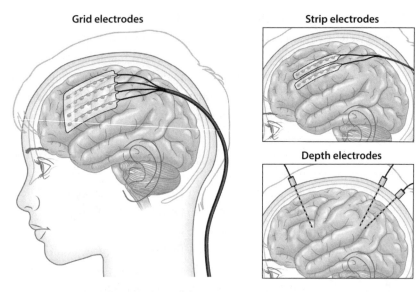

FIGURE 14.1. Invasive monitoring. The figure depicts grid (*left*) and strip (*upper right*) electrodes, which are embedded in thin plastic, surgically implanted, and placed on the surface of the child's brain with wires running to the outside. The figure also (*lower right*) depicts depth electrodes: multiple electrodes that are embedded on a wire and surgically implanted into the brain. In each case, brain electricity is recorded by an EEG machine. The electrodes can also be used for stimulating the underlying brain to localize specific functions.

monitoring unit. Another option is to perform stereoelectroencephalography (stereo EEG). This is a procedure in which depth electrodes are placed into the brain through tiny burr holes in the skull using computer guidance based on MRI to aim the wires at areas of the brain to evaluate. This is very well tolerated by kids and helps the team be sure where seizures are coming from—resective surgery is then done at a later time based on this information.

In some cases, we will have enough information after phase I monitoring to recommend moving forward with surgery. In other cases, the monitoring may determine that surgery is not an option for your child, but recommendations for other treatments may be considered.

In considering whether surgery is the right choice for each patient, we always think about the risks and the benefits. We believe that decisions about surgery require working through a series of questions.

1. Is the child (or the adult) having seizures?

2. Are the seizures recurrent and difficult to control?

3. Are the seizures coming from one location?

4. Can the source of the seizures be easily removed?

If the answer to these four questions is yes, then the next step is to obtain more information. What are the risks of the operation? Is there a risk of losing some motor function, language function, vision, or intellect? What are the potential benefits of the surgery? Is the procedure likely to eliminate the seizures or reduce their frequency? Will it improve the child's quality of life? How much? In what way?

These are only some of the thoughts and concerns you should discuss with your child's physician as you progress toward making decisions about a surgical treatment.

Discussion of the possibility of surgery and its risks and benefits should be an ongoing process. When a focus and its location have been identified, surgery can become a more serious consideration, and a more detailed discussion of its risks and benefits is then possible. The risks will depend on the area to be removed.

As with any operation, there is, of course, a risk of major complications of anesthesia or even death. While the consequences of anesthetic complication can be great, the chances of it occurring are in the range of less than one per one thousand. Infection is also always a risk; so is bleeding or clotting of a blood vessel. All these are potentially serious and capable of causing additional brain damage. Fortunately, these complications occur infrequently. You should ask your child's neurosurgeon about their experience of them.

What are the benefits of epilepsy surgery? The maximum benefit would be freedom from seizures, freedom from taking antiseizure medicine, and freedom from neurological deficit. This is everyone's goal. What are the chances that the goal will be achieved? Surprisingly, it is difficult to give numerical answers to this question. Surgical centers often quote 60–75 percent "good outcomes." This means that perhaps 50 percent of those undergoing an operation will be cured of their seizures, another 10–25 percent will have substantial decrease in the frequency of their seizures, and about 25 percent—one in four—will not be helped.

You cannot, however, apply these statistical figures to your child. Your child's chance of success will depend on the cause of the seizures and the exact location of the focus. The figures quoted also depend on how specific centers select patients for surgery. If they select only ideal candidates, their success rate will be higher. If they take some of the more difficult patients, they may be less "successful," statistically. Your child is unique, and therefore, the discussion and the chances of success are unique. Recent advances in evaluation techniques may have made your child's chances of having a successful outcome better than the published statistics.

In calculating the statistical chances of successful surgery, it is important to differentiate between surgery to remove a lesion (or tumor) and surgery to remove an *epileptic region*. Epilepsy usually comes from the area immediately surrounding a lesion, and a lesion is more easily identified and removed. An epileptic region is more subtle, has less identifiable margins, and, therefore, is more difficult to remove completely. The success rate for surgery to remove lesions causing epilepsy is far higher than that for surgery to remove epileptic regions. In general, the latter surgery is more successful when more tissue is removed.

Whether the risks of surgery are worth the possible benefits is a personal decision. The possibility of being free of seizures will have different value to different people. The risks each individual and family are willing to take to achieve that condition are also very personal. It is our belief, however, that in general, physicians and surgeons have been far too conservative in recommending surgery. Temporal lobe removal may be preferable to taking medication for a lifetime, even if the medication is controlling the seizures with minimal side effects. The anterior part of the temporal lobe on either side may be removed, usually without causing neurological problems. Much of the frontal lobe on either side can also be safely removed, although frontal lobe surgery is typically less successful.

Because language function is usually in the more posterior part of the left frontal and temporal lobes, surgery that might involve that area requires careful evaluation, to weigh the possible risks and benefits. Similarly, since motor function is in the posterior frontal lobe, consideration of surgery near that area also requires careful thought.

When making decisions about surgery, it is your responsibility to look for an epilepsy center that is equipped to evaluate your child properly. Such an epilepsy center should have not only the proper equipment but also the proper team and the proper experience. The best way to find out how capable a center's staff are is to ask them questions. They should not mind your inquiries; in fact, they should encourage them. They should also be happy to put you in touch with other families who have been through this same difficult process—people who realize what kind of a challenging position you are in. They should be willing to have you communicate with families who perhaps have had less than ideal outcomes. You need realistic experiences to make this difficult decision. That doesn't mean that you can or should expect your child to experience the same outcomes or problems. No one can predict this for you. But you should be as informed as you need to be. And remember, this is a potential opportunity for changing the trajectory of your child's seizures and life.

• Feel free to ask how many children with your child's type of seizures they have evaluated.

• Does the center have a team approach? Do the epileptologists work with the surgeons in deciding about the surgery and its boundaries? Is there an epilepsy nurse or social worker who can help you and your child prepare for the evaluation? Is there a neuropsychologist who carefully evaluates each child and follows up with the children after the surgery? In other words, is the team carefully evaluating the outcome of their procedures? Are they as available in the postop evaluation as they have been in the preop considerations?

• Ask about the surgeon's experience. How many similar cases has he or she handled? What were the outcomes?

• Are there other children who have undergone the evaluation? Have they had the surgery? Can you and your child meet them? Can you talk with them about what it was like?

Surgery on the brain is scary. You and your child should enter the decision-making process as partners with your child's physicians, and you and your child should be well informed and comfortable with your decisions and with your epilepsy team.

If surgery is recommended to treat seizures, there are a few different types of surgery to consider.

Focal resection. This is when a specific, relatively small, area of the brain is found to be the seizure onset zone, and it is determined that the benefit of removing the area outweighs the risk (Figure 14.2). For example, there may be an area that didn't form correctly (focal cortical

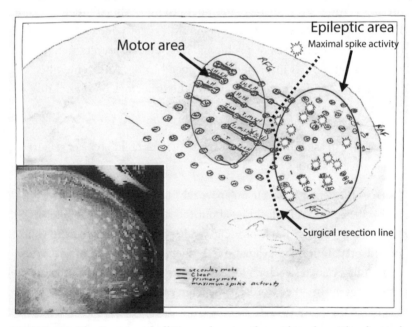

FIGURE 14.2. The inset is a skull X-ray showing the grid in place. The electrodes are visible. Our map of the cortex shows the areas of seizure discharges and the areas of motor activity located by stimulation. The dotted line is the guide for the surgeon to follow in removing the frontal cortex (the epileptic area) and avoiding the motor areas.

dysplasia) in the frontal lobe, and this can be taken out with relatively little risk.

Laser ablation. This is when a laser is used to "burn" or destroy the area that is causing the seizures. Another name for this is LiTT (laser interstitial thermal therapy). A small opening in the skull is made under the guidance of a sophisticated MRI, and the laser probe is placed. This procedure is most common in the setting of mesial temporal sclerosis (scarring of the area containing the amygdala and hippocampus) and is also used in other areas of the brain to treat small tumors or areas of epileptogenicity. There is much less recovery time with this treatment option than a surgery that involves a larger opening of the skull.

Hemispherectomy/Hemispherotomy. This surgery is done when one whole side of the brain is abnormal and causing seizures. In this case the damaged side is disconnected from the good side, and portions of that side of the brain are completely removed.

If there is not a specific area of the brain that can be removed to treat seizures, other surgical options can be used to reduce seizure burden. These include palliative invasive surgeries of tissue (expected to help but not eliminate seizures) and devices.

Palliative Surgical Options

Corpus callosotomy. This surgery cuts the fibers in the corpus callosum deep inside the brain that connect one side of the brain to the other. This surgery is often used for atonic (drop) seizures to prevent serious falls with injury. Corpus callosotomy typically reduces seizures, often by changing the nature and severity of them, but rarely eliminates them.

Multiple subpial transection (MST). The goal of MST is to cut the fibers that are leading to transmission of seizures to other parts of the brain without affecting function in the brain. This surgery is not often performed today, compared to many years ago, but may be returning to popularity due to some recent research.

Resective surgery, removing portions of the brain, can also be palliative. In these cases, some of the seizure focus may be removed, purposely leaving areas that may be more dangerous to resect with the goal of reducing but not eliminating seizures.

Devices

Vagus Nerve Stimulator

The vagus nerve stimulator (VNS) is a small battery-powered device that is implanted under the skin, typically in the left upper chest. A wire goes from the battery to the nerve in the neck called the vagus nerve. It is typically programmed individually in terms of how much current is delivered as well as the frequency and duration of the stimulus. A typical setting delivers current every 5 minutes for 30 seconds, and over time, this stimulation often reduces seizure frequency. It is uncommon for seizures to go away completely with the VNS, but it can often make them better. Most of the time, children need to stay on their antiseizure medicines even with a VNS. An additional benefit is that it does not have the same side effects as medicine. The most common side effect is noticing a hoarse voice when the device is firing. Other side effects such as cough when the device fires can typically be fixed by adjusting the settings on the device.

Newer models of the VNS also detect rapid increases in heart rate, which can indicate the onset of a seizure. When it detects this, it can fire an additional time in attempts to stop a seizure in its tracks. There is also an option to swipe a magnet over the battery when a seizure is occurring. For some patients, swiping a magnet during a seizure will stop the seizure.

The VNS does not work immediately. It takes about 2 months to see any effect after it is put in, but it can continue to have increased benefit for up to 2 years after it is placed. It is therefore important to be patient and wait to see effects after getting a VNS. Over time, on average, 50 percent of patients have a 50 percent improvement in their seizures.

The battery portion of the VNS needs to be replaced about every 7–10 years.

The VNS has also been shown to help with depression, and patients often report feeling better when they have it.

Responsive Neurostimulator

The responsive neurostimulator (RNS, NeuroPace) is a device used if the area of the brain where seizures are starting cannot be safely removed without causing a problem (loss of speech or motor function) or if seizures are starting in multiple areas in the brain.

With this device, electrodes are placed either into or on top of the seizure focus, and these electrodes detect when a seizure is starting and then stimulate (deliver a small electrical current to the brain) in attempts to stop the seizure before it spreads. The battery for this device is placed in a pocket created in the skull. The battery currently needs to be replaced about every 5–6 years, but newer models are extending battery life.

Like the VNS, the RNS takes some adjustment to the settings over time and becomes more effective as it is in place longer.

There are no head-to-head studies comparing VNS to RNS; however, in general the VNS has been shown to reduce seizures about 40–50 percent in 50 percent of people after 2 years and rarely leads to seizure freedom. RNS, when used in an identified seizure focus, has been shown to lead to a 50 percent reduction in seizures in about 70 percent of patients in a period of 6 months, and to seizure freedom in 20 percent of patients. It is less successful when the seizure focus is not clear. Right now, this is not formally approved in children, but many centers are getting it covered by insurance companies if the situation is appropriate. A multi-center trial that we hope will lead to approval is underway in teenagers. It can't be used in the youngest of patients because the skull is not thick enough to support the device and the skull hasn't stopped growing.

Deep Brain Stimulation

The deep brain stimulator (DBS, Percept) is a device that is also used to treat intractable epilepsy. Electrodes are placed into the thalamus (deep gray matter structure of the brain), and settings are adjusted for stimulation of this brain area to reduce seizure frequency.

While the wires for this device are in the thalamus, the battery is placed under the skin of the chest or abdomen.

Over time the DBS can decrease the severity of seizures and decrease frequency of seizures by up to 50–60 percent, and this result also seems to improve over time. It is unlikely to completely eliminate seizures. Some side effects reported have been a negative effect on mood and memory. It is also not approved in children at this time.

Getting a Second Opinion

If your child is seeing a neurologist in a center that does not perform epilepsy surgery, your child's physician should be able to give you the names of several centers specializing in epilepsy and epilepsy surgery. Most physicians will be understanding if you seek a second opinion and will provide you with your child's records. In addition, you can begin doing research yourself by looking at the Epilepsy Foundation or the National Association of Epilepsy Centers (NAEC) websites and talking with other parents. These are just some of the ways you can get the names of epilepsy centers. You should call the center and ask pertinent questions about their programs: How frequently do they do epilepsy surgery? In what age ranges? With what success rates? You will find that most centers will want to do their own monitoring, even though it may have been done recently elsewhere. This is perfectly reasonable, since the interpretation of the monitoring is the basis for deciding how to proceed. Centers such as ours review all the child's records prior to making an appointment to see the child, so that we can have the most cost-effective visit with the parent and child.

Finding the right place to do the surgery can be complicated. Different centers perform different surgeries, and there is often a waiting list for all of them. Remember, this isn't an emergency. Do not make the mistake of choosing a center on the basis of who can do the operation soonest. *There is not just one center for epilepsy surgery in the United States, nor just one surgeon.*

Unfortunately, in this era of managed care, not all patients are able to go to the center of their choice, because of the constraints of insurance. (Insurance issues are discussed in Chapter 21.) It is important to recognize that epilepsy surgery, and all the preliminary evaluation and follow-up care, is very expensive. Out-of-network costs can escalate rapidly, leaving a family with an overwhelming mountain of bills. No one should have to sell their home, move to another city, or go to extremes to be able to have surgery for their child. Most epilepsy programs can recommend a center for the surgery that is within your network. The evaluation for epilepsy surgery is a long and tedious process. If traveling great distances is a limiting factor, a center can be found near where you live. Most centers are willing to help you find the place that will be able to meet your needs and those of your child.

Deciding to Pursue Surgery

While each step in the process of evaluating a child for surgery requires careful thought, the conclusion of the invasive (phase II) monitoring, when all available information has been collected, is when we decide exactly what we recommend be done during surgery and reconsider the potential risks and benefits. We accomplish this with a meeting of the whole team that has been involved in the evaluation. This team includes the epilepsy specialist who has been your child's primary physician, our group of monitoring specialists, those who have carefully assessed language and intellectual function, the counselor who has been working closely with the child and the family, and the surgeon who will be performing the operation. At this conference we carefully assess where the seizures appear to be coming from, what surgery can be done to eliminate them, what normal functions might be damaged by the surgery, and other potential risks and benefits of the procedure. At times we decide that surgery should not be performed. After the group reaches consensus, we then present our opinions to the patient and family, who must independently decide whether to proceed with surgery and whether their perception of the risks and benefits is similar to ours.

The family's considerations regarding surgery are different from those of the epilepsy team. It is the epilepsy team's responsibility to evaluate whether surgery is feasible and what the medical and physical risks of the surgery are likely to be. The team can also assess the likelihood of seizure control. The value of these benefits to you and your child and the acceptability of the risks must be determined by you and your child. Epilepsy surgery is rarely an emergency. There is time to think carefully about the decision, to seek second opinions, and to talk with patients who have undergone the proposed surgery. Sometimes the team's assessment of the risks and benefits may not be the same as the patient's or the family's. In that situation, it is important to sit down and explore these differences to come to a satisfactory decision. We have often found it useful to have parents who are anticipating surgery meet with families and children who have previously undergone a similar procedure. It is impossible to conceptualize what a child who has undergone a hemispherectomy (disconnection of half the brain) will be like without seeing and talking with such a child.

There is sometimes a disparity between how the two parents see the problem of their child's seizures and how they feel about the risks and potential benefits of surgery. At visits long before the surgery, we discuss with both parents the need for agreement. We emphasize that a child's parents, even parents who are not together, must be in agreement before we will proceed. If something goes wrong at surgery, or if the surgery is unsuccessful, we do not ever want one parent to be blaming the other. We often tell parents, "Every morning hereafter you will have to get up and look yourself in the mirror while you shave or comb your hair. If the surgery goes well, as it usually does, you will smile and say, 'I only wish that we had done it sooner.' But, if things go badly—if your child has complications, if they are worse off than before the surgery, or if they die (and that is a remote possibility)—you still have to face yourself in that mirror every day and be able to say, 'We made the best decision for our child that we knew how to make.' "

Including the Child in the Decision

Children are often left out of the decision-making process. Depending on their age and their level of function, however, they should be included. Older children should participate in the decision to do surgery. They must understand the probable outcomes of the procedure. Meeting another child who has had surgery may help them assess the situation. Unless the child and both parents agree to the surgery, surgery should not be performed.

Tips for Parents of Children Undergoing Invasive Monitoring or Surgery

If your child is old enough to understand, be sure that you have prepared them well for the hospitalization and for the procedure. The unknown is always more frightening than something that has been explained.

Monitoring

Prior to the monitoring, you should have a discussion with the staff on the monitoring unit. You should ask:

• What is the room like?

• Is my child allowed to move about the room?

• What clothes should we bring?

• What toys and videos may we bring? What will they have on the unit? Will there be a good internet connection?

• How will the electrodes be placed?

Monitoring is a boring time for the child.

• Bring a bag of inexpensive "surprises." Games, toys, books, and snacks can be wrapped ahead of time. Each day allow the child to pick one as a reward for having done well that day. We call these incentives, not bribes.

• Depending on the age, bring a favorite stuffed animal or two and a favorite blanket.

• Bring clothes and pajamas that don't pull over the head.

Monitoring is an anxious time for parents. Some common questions asked by parents are:

• Will my child have enough seizures for the monitoring to be useful?

• If they reduce the medications, will my child have too many seizures? Will they have status epilepticus?

• How long will it take to get "enough" seizures? How many is enough?

• Will they get enough seizures and be able to operate?

Don't be afraid to ask these and other questions before and during the monitoring.

Surgery

If surgery is planned, preparing the child and the rest of the family (siblings included) is essential. No matter how calm your child may seem on the outside, on the inside, the child (not to mention siblings, and you, the parents) is frightened. Appropriately so!

Sometimes presurgical counseling is useful for the child and for siblings. Ask your child's neurologist or neurosurgeon if they can help. Talking with other families and children who have been through the surgical procedure can be invaluable. Ask them how they felt. Ask how they dealt with specific problems. Ask what problems to anticipate. Ask for practical tips. Most parents are delighted and eager to share their experiences, both the good and the bad, and even their most personal feelings. We have found that our parent support network is one of our greatest assets. Every parent benefits from those who have gone before, and everyone is willing to help those who will come after. Older children are also willing to share their experiences with an individual of a similar age. Both children derive benefit.

For *some* children, particularly teenage girls, the most traumatic part of the surgery may be having to have their head shaved. In many cases, only a very small amount of hair needs to be shaved, so it is important to talk to your child's neurosurgeon about this to allay this fear.

The Hospital Routine for Patients Undergoing Surgery

Every hospital has a different routine, and surgeons have different preferences. We are going to present the Hopkins routine for you as an example, but be sure to ask about the timelines and routines at the hospital where your child is having surgery.

• Our children usually have a preoperative evaluation before surgery. They will be checked for infection, and blood will be drawn to check for bleeding and clotting abnormalities and for cross-matching. The child and the parents will see the neurologist and/or the neurosurgeon to answer any last-minute questions that any of them may have.

• Instructions are given about eating and drinking on the morning of the surgery, as well as where and when to report for surgery.

• The anticipated duration of the surgery, and why it takes so long, is also discussed. We explain that it takes time to put the child to sleep, to put in all the appropriate intravenous lines, and to shave the head and prepare the scalp. Often, two hours have elapsed before the operation even begins.

• Nurses or physicians come out of the operating room from time to time to update the parents on the progress of the surgery.

• When the surgery is completed, it may take one to two hours to put everything back together—to make sure that the wound is completely secured and that wires are carefully identified and securely wrapped.

Most of the time the child is in the operating room is spent getting the child ready for the operation and closing after the operation. The time you spend waiting only seems to last forever.

After surgery, children may go to the ICU (intensive care unit) recovery room, where they will be monitored closely.

• We tell parents how much time will elapse before the child will be transferred from the ICU or recovery room to the epilepsy monitoring unit or to the less intensive care floor, depending on the surgery performed.

• We warn parents to expect the child's eyes to be swollen and to expect them to have headaches, which we medicate.

• We try to prepare parents for the worst, since they are then relieved when it is not so bad.

• We warn families that when the doctors come around to check on the child, they often do not linger, and that therefore parents should write down their list of questions so that they will remember to ask them. Under the stresses of the surgery and the postoperative period, questions can easily be forgotten.

We also tell parents to have discussions with the child's school administrators and teachers and with the other students so that they all will know about the surgery and what to expect when the child returns to class with a funny looking haircut and a scar. If the other children know, they can be supportive.

Postoperative care depends on many factors, particularly the type of surgery that was done. It will typically vary from minimal needs, if the surgery involved only implanting electrodes for stereoelectroencephalography, for example, to possibly considerably more issues if a large resection was undertaken. Prior to surgery, postop plans should be discussed on a preliminary basis. If significant rehabilitation might be necessary, it is important to know what resources are available and how they will affect your family (proximity to home, etc.).

PART IV

Practical Issues
OF Living WITH
Epilepsy

CHAPTER 15

Routine Medical Care and Epilepsy

We are frequently called by parents, physicians, and dentists for advice about whether a medical procedure can be done safely on a child with seizures. They may be frightened by the potential effects of antiseizure medications (ASMs) or intimidated by the thought of a seizure occurring during the procedure or while the child is under anesthesia.

Since anesthesia is the ultimate treatment for uncontrollable seizures, general anesthesia, used for an operation, typically will not cause seizures. The anesthesiologist must consider the child's epilepsy in choosing the medications to be used for the procedure, and the child should be monitored carefully. The anesthesiologist must also be aware of possible interactions between their anesthetic and the ASMs the child is taking. In addition, if a child with epilepsy requires anesthesia, a major concern is the inability of the child to receive his standard ASM by mouth. If the child is to receive nothing by mouth (NPO) for 12 to 24 hours, it is advisable to give an extra dose of their regular medication prior to surgery. Routinely, pediatric anesthesiologists recommend that children take their regular medications, with just a sip of water, on the morning prior to surgery. If the child cannot receive anything by mouth for a long period after surgery, intravenous ASM may be necessary. It is important to discuss this in advance because some ASMs do not have intravenous formulations.

Q. *"Can my child be put to sleep for dental care?"*
A. Yes. The standard anesthetics used for dental care will neither in-

crease the likelihood of seizures nor affect the ASM's effectiveness. Some children continue to have seizures despite medication. Anyone performing a procedure on such a child should be capable of managing the seizure just as the parent would do at home.

Q. *"Is there anything different that should be done for the child who has epilepsy and requires anesthesia?"*
A. No. If a child should have a generalized seizure, they will require an open airway. Therefore, posterior nasal packing (packing the back of the nose with gauze, to stop bleeding), sometimes done after a tonsillectomy or adenoidectomy, should be done with considerable caution and careful observation postoperatively.

Q. *"What about cold medicines and cough syrups?"*
A. Antihistamines and decongestants have been reported to decrease seizure threshold. It appears to us that some children may be quite sensitive to these medications. We have no ability to identify which children will react with a seizure when given these over-the-counter drugs. There is no evidence that these medications actually alter the cold or flu; they merely ease the symptoms. It is said that a cold well treated lasts seven days; poorly treated, a week. So maybe just skipping these symptomatic medicines would be best. A parent could also consider using a saline nose spray to relieve a stuffy nose and help clear a nasal discharge.

If you feel that it is necessary to give your child one of the medications because the symptoms are very severe, and then your child has a seizure, the seizure may have been precipitated by the cold medicine. On the other hand, it may have been precipitated by the illness. Or again, it could be coincidental. If your child repeatedly has seizures after receiving one of these medications, it would be prudent not to use them.

Q. *"Are there any other medications that my child should not receive?"*
A. Stimulants such as dextroamphetamine (Dexedrine) and methylphenidate (Ritalin) are often useful managing attention deficit hyperactivity disorder. Although in the large doses occasionally used for psychiatric conditions (and in some animal models), these drugs have been re-

ported to precipitate seizures, there is no consistent evidence that they have an adverse effect in children with epilepsy. When needed, their benefits clearly outweigh any potential risks.

Q. *"Are vitamins and supplements beneficial?"*
A. Except in the rare individual who has a documented vitamin deficiency, there is no evidence that vitamins are beneficial (or detrimental) in treating epilepsy. Always make your child's physician aware of any supplements you are considering giving to your child.

Q. *"Can my child receive routine immunizations?"*
A. Yes, children with seizures and epilepsy can and should receive their immunizations, even the pertussis immunization. There may be a slight reaction to some vaccines, which may cause a fever, and that fever may be enough to precipitate a seizure, but there is no evidence that current immunizations either cause epilepsy or make epilepsy worse. There is also no evidence that immunizations cause permanent encephalopathy.

Nonetheless, when a young child has just begun to have seizures and the physician has not yet determined the cause of the epilepsy, and that child has worsening seizures or a change in their development rate after an immunization, then parents are often convinced that the immunization caused the child's problems to get worse. It is often easier to defer the immunization for a few months until the course of the epilepsy and of the child's development becomes clearer. Then that child can be immunized. It is very clear that the immunizations currently recommended by the Academy of Pediatrics are far safer for the child than the diseases they are designed to prevent.

Q. *"Can my child take antibiotics while on ASMs?"*
Q. *"Roberta developed a sore throat yesterday, and her pediatrician started her on an antibiotic. Roberta is allergic to penicillin, so he put her on something called erythromycin. Today I can barely wake her up, and she seems drunk. Do you think that this erythromycin is too strong for her?"*
A. Roberta is on carbamazepine (Tegretol) for her seizures. Erythromycin interferes with the metabolism of carbamazepine and makes the

blood level go very high. When a child on carbamazepine is given erythromycin, one must reduce the amount of carbamazepine by one-third. When the antibiotic is stopped, go back to the original dose.

Whenever a child is on an ASM and a new medication of any kind is given, ask your child's physician or pharmacist if the new drug has any interactions with the old one.

CHAPTER 16

Comorbidities

Other Problems that Can Co-occur with Epilepsy

"Will my children have problems learning?"

"Are my child's mood and attention problems due to their epilepsy?"

People used to think that issues with learning, thinking, behavior, or mood in children with epilepsy were caused by the seizures, by medications, or by the child's adjustment to having epilepsy. Certainly, these things can contribute to a child's difficulties, but they are not always the cause. We now know that the same underlying factors causing the brain to be prone to seizures are likely causing the brain to be prone to some other co-occurring conditions we sometimes see.

The specific areas of strength and weakness in children and adolescents with epilepsy depends on multiple factors, such as seizure type, seizure frequency, the underlying brain condition, medication effects, and genetic predispositions.

Let us reassure you first that:

• most children with epilepsy have normal intelligence.

• most children with epilepsy do not have problems with thinking, learning, mood, behavior, or social skills.

You should also remember that many children without epilepsy have problems of various kinds. Thus, even if your child does have problems, they may not be related to epilepsy itself.

Developmental Delays

As children develop and grow, their motor, speech, and cognitive development follow a predictable sequence. While there is a range of "normal" in terms of time frames, *developmental delay* is when your child does not reach their developmental milestones in the expected time range.

Some children with epilepsy can experience developmental delays due to the underlying brain condition, the seizures themselves, medications, or limitations in opportunity to engage in typical developmental activities.

The term developmental "delay" is misleading, as it implies a child will "catch up." What it often means is that a child will continue to make developmental gains over their lifetime, but their overall abilities will likely remain behind peers at each age. It is also rather nonspecific since it doesn't describe more clearly what area of development seems delayed or impaired.

It's also important to realize that children with significant neurological conditions may not follow the same predictable sequence of development or may have atypical patterns of development. For example, a child who experienced an early stroke may always walk with a limp due to weakness. Because of this, assigning a "developmental age" to a child may not capture the individual strengths, weaknesses, abilities, and challenges unique to that particular child.

Sometimes a child is diagnosed with developmental delay early on, before the individual child's developmental trajectory is clear. Clinicians are sometimes hesitant to diagnose conditions such as intellectual disability or cerebral palsy in young children with cognitive or motor abilities that are below peers until they are older and the developmental progression is clearer, particularly if they have other medical conditions. Similarly, the coding of "developmental delay" for school services can be used only at younger ages and must be changed to another coding if the child continues to require special education (currently in 2021, this must happen after age 7). This is to define and describe the nature of the problem more clearly.

Cerebral Palsy

Cerebral palsy (CP) is a condition in which the brain's control of motor movements or posture is abnormal. It is caused by damage within the motor areas of the brain or spinal cord that has occurred before or during birth or early childhood. It is not caused by a tumor or by degeneration of the nervous system. CP is not progressive—it does not continue to become worse—although it may become more obvious, or its symptoms may vary slightly as the child matures.

Q. *"Will my child who has cerebral palsy be intellectually disabled?"*
A. About half of children with cerebral palsy are intellectually disabled to some degree; a number of others may have behavioral and learning problems. Some have no such problems and are of normal intelligence; indeed, some children with CP have superior intelligence.

Epilepsy is quite common in children with CP and depends on what caused the cerebral palsy in the first place, but few children with epilepsy will have CP. Epilepsy does not cause cerebral palsy; it does not cause intellectual disability. Nor does cerebral palsy cause epilepsy. When CP and epilepsy do occur together, underlying damage to the brain has caused both.

Types of Cerebral Palsy

Many classification systems are in use, and they generally depend on who is using them. One important factor is how severe the problem is. This ranges from mild, when the child can move through their daily activities without any assistance, to severe, when the child requires a wheelchair. Neurologists and orthopedists are typically more concerned about what parts of the body are involved, what kind of movement or muscle problems exist, and what the nature of the muscle tone is. If we're concerned about the part of the body and extent of the involvement, you would hear the terms *paresis* (weakened) or *plegic* (paralyzed), as well as *mono* (one limb), *hemi* (half the body—one side), *para* (lower part of the body), or perhaps quadriplegia, where all four limbs are affected. We would also talk about motor function, whether there is constant increased muscle tone or whether the movements are fluctuating. Spastic cerebral palsy would mean that tone was always increased. Motor function might also be described as either *pyramidal*, which involves particular nerve fibers, or *extrapyramidal*, which means that certain parts of the brain, like the basal ganglia, thalamus, or cerebellum, are involved. The latter usually indicates an abnormality of the type of movement. It could be *ataxic* (affecting balance and coordination), *athetoid* (slow, writhing involuntary movements), *dystonic* (twisted postures), or *chorea* (irregular, jerky, shaking movements).

A child with a hemiparesis and difficult-to-control seizures on the paralyzed side should be evaluated for possible epilepsy surgery by an epilepsy center. Seizures due to early strokes or to developmental abnormalities of the brain may be very difficult to control with any combination of ASMs. Surgery to remove the affected portion of the brain may give that child the best chance for seizure control and for more normal function without medication. When such a child has not responded to the first two medications, that may be the time to consider a surgical evaluation.

Sarah was 5 years old, a bright young lady with a congenital left hemiparesis. She was 5 months old when it was first noted that she was not using her left arm. She was diagnosed as having delayed development and cerebral palsy. A CT scan and later an MRI scan showed evidence of a stroke in her right cortex caused by a thrombosis (blood clot) in the right middle cerebral artery. At 4 years of age, she had her first seizure; it was status epilepticus. Over the next few months, she had more generalized seizures despite several different medications, and she developed myoclonic jerks and drop spells so that she could barely stand or walk. She was tried on the ketogenic diet and did well for several months, but the seizures broke through.

The family finally agreed to a right hemispherectomy to remove the whole damaged area. Sarah was 10 and in the third grade in a regular class at the time of this photo. She walks, runs, and plays with her classmates, wearing a short leg brace. She uses her left hand only as a helper

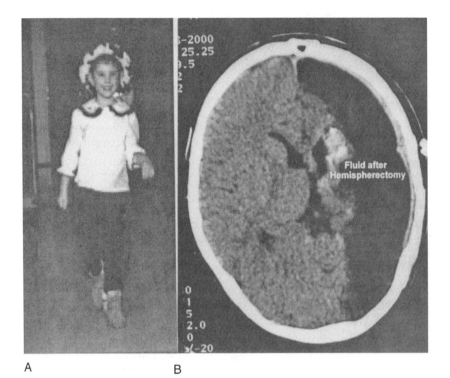

A   B

FIGURE 16.1. (A) Sarah after hemispherectomy. Note the posturing of her left arm as she walks. (B) An MRI scan of Sarah's head shows the intact left hemisphere. Fluid has filled in where the other hemisphere was removed.

hand. Physically she is no different than she was prior to surgery, but she has had no seizures in those three years and was on no medication (Figure 16.1).

Intellectual Disability

Most children have "normal" intelligence; the "average" intelligence quotient (IQ) is given the number 100, and 95 percent of children have IQs between 70 and 130. While there are many questions and much debate about the meaning of an IQ score and about the tests by which it is determined, in a rough way, it is shorthand for overall cognitive ability. Most children with epilepsy have IQ scores within the normal range. If psychologists look at the range and distribution of the IQ scores for a large number of children with epilepsy, however, they find a larger than expected number with scores in the low-normal range. This is not because of the epilepsy itself, but usually because of what has caused the epilepsy. If the child had meningitis or a stroke or problems with the brain's development, then those problems could have both affected the child's intelligence and caused the epilepsy.

Intellectual disability (ID) is a term used when there are limits to a person's ability to learn at an expected level and function in daily life. Intellectual disability was formerly called *mental retardation*, but that term is no longer used. IDs are defined as neurodevelopmental disorders that begin in childhood and are characterized by intellectual difficulties as well as difficulties in conceptual, social, and practical areas of daily living. Deficits in both adaptive functioning (level of independence) and intellectual functioning (reasoning, problem solving, planning, abstract thinking, judgment, academic learning, and learning from experience) are required for the diagnosis and need to be confirmed by clinical evaluation and individualized standard IQ testing. While there is no cutoff for diagnosis, typically IQ and adaptive skills more than two standard deviations below age expectations (below 70 on an IQ or adaptive measure) is considered in the range of intellectual disability. The current diagnostic criteria are based on the *Diagnostic and Statistical Manual of Mental Disorders, 5th Edition (DSM-5)*.

Intellectual disability can be caused by a problem that starts any time before a child turns 18 years old—even before birth. It can be caused by injury, disease, or a problem in the brain. For many children, the cause of their intellectual disability is not known. Intelligence is the result of many factors. The intelligence of parents and the environment in which the child is raised are the most important.

One factor to consider, if your child is having difficulties in school, is their IQ. If their IQ is toward the lower end of the normal range, learning to read or doing math may be more difficult for them than for the rest of the class. The frustration associated with these difficulties could cause behavioral problems and acting out. Since these problems might be easily solved by a different class placement or by special help, it is important to recognize their cause early. Knowledge of your child's intelligence might also change your expectations and those of their teachers, removing undue pressure.

A bright child, in a class that is beneath their abilities, may also be bored and not do the work or might act out. So, occasionally, a child's school problems are because the child is too smart for the class and requires more challenge.

One wonderful first-grader was referred to us by his teacher because he was having difficulties reading and was not participating in class. The teacher wanted him tested. His parents couldn't understand, since he had no reading problems at home, only at school. A few questions to his family revealed that his favorite activity at home was actually reading *Popular Mechanics* and trying to build some of the things he found there. His response to the school problem was "I don't care about *Ramona the Pest*. It's for babies." This young man clearly did not have a reading problem or a learning problem. He had a classroom boredom problem.

Medications may also affect a child's performance in school and on IQ tests.

Learning Problems

Intelligence is only one of the critical factors in a child's ability to learn. For example, reading is a complex task. The child must first see the letters, and the seeing must then be translated into electrical signals in the eye. These signals are then sent to the occipital lobe of the brain, the area that is responsible for the primary processing of visual information. From there the message goes to the association areas of the brain in the parietal lobe, where the symbols are interpreted. Meaning comes from association with something that the child remembers, memories that must be retrieved from the frontal and temporal lobes.

Children and adolescents with epilepsy have been shown to be at increased risk for academic difficulties. Early identification of a problem, if it exists, can assist in the development of strategies for compensation and lead to a far more successful school experience. Yet, learning problems can also be secondary to medication, to psychological stress, and to the school's and the teacher's reaction to the child and to epilepsy.

Problems with reading could occur at many levels. A child with vision problems, who needs glasses, may not be able to see the letters. A child with damage in the occipital lobes might have normal eyes but might not "see" the letters. One with dysfunction in the association areas of the brain might be able to see the letters but might not be able to recognize them. Problems in other areas might keep them from being able to retrieve the memories that give the words meaning.

These varied difficulties with reading often go under the heading of *dyslexia*. *Dys* means not working properly, and *lexia* means having to do with words. In most children the basic cause of the dyslexia is not understood, but we do know that dyslexia is more common in children who have a family member with dyslexia and is more common in some neurological conditions.

You may hear physicians and psychologists use the terms dyslexia, dyscalculia, and dysgraphia to refer to problems in reading, math, or writing. In school and special education settings, these problems fall under a specific learning disorder or disability (in reading, math, or written language). To meet criteria (based on the *DSM-5*) for a diagnosis of specific learning disorder or disability, the child must have (1) trouble with reading, reading comprehension, spelling, written expression, number concepts, or math reasoning; and (2) academic skills that are substantially below what is expected for the child's age and that cause problems in school, work, or everyday activities. The difficulties can't be due to lack of exposure, or due to something else (like vision or hearing problems, or another disorder). Schools are moving toward a *response to intervention* model, so that a child needs to still have these problems after they are provided with targeted intervention to continue meeting criteria for diagnosis.

Learning by listening is also a multistage process. It involves hearing and paying attention to what is said. It involves transmission of the electrical signals to the association cortex, where they must be recognized and associated with memories and actions. Thus, another type of learning problem might be associated with problems in hearing, attending, word recognition, and the association of words with memories.

Learning by seeing and learning by hearing are but two of the many multistep processes that may pose difficulties with learning. It is rare for anyone to have a complete block in one of these learning channels. More commonly, a child will function poorly in one or more processes, and a learning problem will result. Some children learn better by listening to information, others by reading information. Most children will find their own best learning style. Some children with greater weaknesses in one area will require special help to get around their areas of difficulty and to maximize their strengths.

A child who is having learning problems in school, whether they have epilepsy or not, should be referred to the school's special education team (see Chapter 17) and be evaluated by the school and/or outside providers to identify their strengths and weaknesses and to make recommendations for intervention. Only then will the teachers be able to find the best way to help them learn. For some children, this will mean extra help. Others may require resource teachers with special training. Still others may need to repeat a grade, be placed in a class that moves at a slower pace or attend a special education class or even school. Each child and their struggles are unique. The child must be individually assessed and a plan developed to meet that child's specific needs. All of these statements are true for the child with learning problems, whether or not that child has epilepsy. They are not different for the child with epilepsy; the problems are only more common, or may be more nuanced.

Attention Problems and Hyperactivity

One of the most common problems in children and adolescents with epilepsy is attention. Research suggests that up to 30 percent of children with epilepsy also meet criteria for a diagnosis of attention deficit hyperactivity disorder (ADHD), with the majority best characterized by the inattentive subtype.

To learn, one must pay attention to what is being taught. Teachers know that the attention span of young children is short. Therefore, they teach in short blocks of time interspersed with activities, such as marching around the room or recess. As the child gets older (and the nervous system and attention span mature), the child is able to sit and concentrate or attend for increasingly long periods. A potential cause of a learning problem in the early years of school is that the child's nervous system is not yet sufficiently mature to allow the child to attend for long periods.

Another cause of attention problems could be that the material is too difficult or too easy for the child, causing daydreaming or lack of focus. A child who hasn't eaten and is hungry may also be less likely to pay attention. A child who hasn't had enough sleep may have similar problems. There are many different reasons a child might not pay attention in school.

If attention difficulties are significant enough to interfere with learning, a child may meet criteria for ADHD. Current terminology for this diagnosis uses ADHD with three subtypes: inattentive subtype (which sometimes used to be called attention deficit disorder, or ADD), the hyperactive/impulsive subtype, and the combined subtype. According to the *DSM-5*, to meet criteria for ADHD, a child must demonstrate a persistent pattern of inattention and/or hyperactivity and impulsivity that interferes with functioning or development. This is quantified as six or more symptoms of inattention, and/or six or more symptoms of hyperactivity/impulsivity (as listed in the manual). Specific examples of symptoms are "often has difficulty sustaining attention to tasks or play activities" and "often fails to give close attention to details or makes careless mistakes." Clinicians and psychiatrists use the *DSM-5* to diagnose psychiatric illnesses, and ADHD is considered, in the broadest terms, a psychiatric illness. Clinicians need to use these diagnostic categories to accurately describe a child's problems and for coverage issues (insurance and service provision). ADHD is more common (or more easily recognized) in boys, where overactivity is frequently an accompanying symptom and more likely to draw attention to the child. Attention deficit disorders are not uncommon in children during the early school years; they are perhaps more common in children with epilepsy. They are also frequently associated with "immaturity" of the nervous system and with the learning disorders described above.

Although the cause of ADHD is unknown, we like to think of it as a problem with filtering. Everyone is constantly bombarded by multiple different stimuli. As you are reading this chapter, there may be children playing in the room, the TV blaring, the clock ticking, and someone else talking. And yet you are able to filter out all these other stimuli and concentrate, pay attention to what you are reading. We do not know exactly how this filtering takes place, but it seems to be to be partly a learned skill and partly a result of nervous system maturity. (By the way, did you notice the repetition of the words *to be* in the previous sentence, or weren't you paying attention?) Infants and young children are easily distracted by the many stimuli around them; they have difficulty paying attention. As they get older, they can attend better. Some children mature faster in this respect than others. Some have far more difficulty paying attention than others and are diagnosed as having attention deficit disorders when the problem interferes with their work in school.

Some medications decrease a child's ability to pay attention; others appear to increase the child's ability to attend. Perhaps these drugs act on the filter, either allowing more stimuli to reach consciousness and thus distract or increasing the filtering so that the child is less aware of the distractions and can concentrate better.

Phenobarbital is known to increase the inattentiveness of some children and to cause hyperactivity as well. Other medications, such as topiramate, have also been shown to cause drowsiness and slowed cognition. Some drugs, such as methylphenidate (Ritalin), may act by improving the filter of inattentive (or hyperactive) children, allowing them to concentrate better. They are not contraindicated in children with epilepsy. These medications typically work at the neurotransmitter level, allowing the proper amount of a transmitter to be available for more normal functional activity of the neurons that are needed for focusing attention. There are many new medications for ADHD. A discussion of these medications is beyond the scope of this book.

It's important to monitor whether the medication is actually helping the child in school. Once again, open dialogue with your child's teacher is important. Not all children with learning problems have attention deficit disorder. Not all learning problems are due to medication. Some children with and without medication, and with and without epilepsy, have problems in school. Not all children are the same height and the same weight or have the same learning styles or the same learning capacities. Children should not be treated identically in school; every child has special needs, and every child needs to be treated as an individual to bring out that child's special needs and special assets.

Sometimes all that is required is a bit of creativity. One of our patients was in a very expensive private school. His seizures had been controlled, but he was about to be expelled because he couldn't pass his tests. It turned out that he was smart enough, but he couldn't complete the tests in the allotted time. Arranging for him to take untimed tests showed that he knew the material and had learned what was taught. If a test in school is to see if children have learned the material, why do they have to reproduce it in a fixed time? Ask about untimed tests. Ask about using a computer if writing is a problem. What about oral tests? What about speech to text/text to speech technology for the visually impaired? What about using an audio book for those with reading problems? Creativity can be an answer to many children with learning problems.

When children with epilepsy are having difficulty focusing their attention, we need to ask if their antiseizure medication may be the cause. All antiseizure medications are capable of causing both attention and learning problems. Every parent of a child with epilepsy should be aware of their child's school performance and note if there is a change (for better or worse) when the child is started on medication, when the medication is changed to a new drug, or when the dosage is changed.

If a child has attention problems, school accommodations that may be appropriate include preferential seating away from windows or close to the teacher, frequent breaks and shorter study times, allowing movement or standing if it does not disrupt the class, testing in a separate room, use of a signal for redirection, and, if attention problems are severe, a 1:1 aide or smaller class size may be appropriate.

Anxiety and Mood Issues

Children with epilepsy are at increased risk of mood and psychiatric problems compared with children without epilepsy and those with other chronic illnesses not involving the brain.

Research shows that anywhere from 5 percent to 40 percent of children with epilepsy have anxiety, 12–25 percent of children with epilepsy experience depression, and 5–13 percent of children with epilepsy have a behavioral disorder. We used to think that these co-occurring psychological difficulties were primarily due to consequences of stigmatization, life obstacles, and other psychosocial stressors. The more recent theory in the field, however, is that the shared underlying neurobiological mechanisms responsible for the manifestations of seizures play a large role in these comorbidities.

There is some suggestion that younger age of seizure onset and longer duration of epilepsy have been associated with the presence of anxiety and depressive symptoms. Seizure frequency and severity, as well as being on multiple medications, have also been associated with mood symptoms. Further, focal seizures that start in the temporal and frontal lobes are sometimes associated with increased behavioral problems, anxiety, and depression.

About 4 percent of the general population has generalized anxiety disorder, a constant state of tension or worry. The number is much higher for people with epilepsy. Anxiety disorders have been associated with the amygdala, a structure in the front part of the temporal lobe. Seizures that start in the temporal lobe frequently affect the amygdala and cause it to act in different ways. Anxiety can also be directly related to worrying about the possibility of having another seizure. Not knowing when a seizure may occur can increase worry about having one in an embarrassing or dangerous situation. It is often the possibility of having a seizure, rather than the seizure itself, that handicaps the person with epilepsy. Afraid of having a seizure in public and the real possibility of injury, people with epilepsy may seclude themselves. As a result, they may become isolated. Some children are more susceptible to anxiety disorders. Genetic influences and a person's response to stress may play a part in their development. Women are more likely than men to have anxiety disorders, and patients with psychogenic nonepileptic seizures also have higher rates of anxiety. Anxiety and epilepsy can be so closely linked that seizures are sometimes mistaken for panic attacks in those who have never had seizures before.

All children have times when they are sad or feel upset. It's normal for children to have feelings about their diagnosis of epilepsy or be sad about limitations their seizures may put on their life. For some people, their epilepsy and mood problems are not connected, but potential links may be related to how epilepsy affects their life. Possible side effects of antiseizure medications (ASMs) include mood changes, irritability, agitation, or depression. With some people, however, ASMs can improve their mood.

While the underlying brain condition causing the seizures may be causing mood difficulties, the same treatments for these conditions that work for children without epilepsy are appropriate. You should talk openly to your child about their seizures, and diagnosis of epilepsy, in language that is appropriate for their age. Demystifying the condition and answering questions will reduce the chance that your child will worry or think incorrect things about their epilepsy. Cognitive-behavioral therapy can help children identify thoughts and feelings that lead to anxiety or mood problems, as well as learn strategies to reduce stress and use positive self-talk.

Behavior

Roughly one in four children with epilepsy has significant behavioral problems. Another one in four has emotional difficulties that are less severe but still disturbing. In general, behavioral problems are more troublesome in children whose seizures began at an early age. This is especially true for boys, who are more likely to act out, but girls are also affected. Their emotional problems may be recognized less often.

You may suspect that your child's behavioral problems are related to the epilepsy itself. It is true that behavioral difficulties can be caused or worsened by epilepsy. Several aspects of epilepsy can affect the brain and contribute to behavioral problems, including the underlying brain condition, the seizures themselves, possible electrical discharges between seizures, and medication effects. Any of these can impair normal brain functions or may cause chemical imbalances in the brain that lead to psychiatric difficulties. In some cases, small effects accumulate over many years and cause psychiatric problems to emerge in adulthood.

You may see brief periods of abnormal behavior leading up to a seizure, during a seizure, or for a few days following a seizure. A few children swing back and forth between uncontrolled seizures and bad behavior.

If we think of seizures as caused by misfiring neurons, or inefficient brain networks, it's not surprising that children with seizures are prone to dysregulated behavior, impulsivity, lack of inhibition, and aggression or outbursts. Behavioral disorders, also known as disruptive behavioral disorders, are the most common reasons that parents are told to take their children for mental health assessments and treatment. It's import-ant to remember that even if the epilepsy or neurological condition is an explanation for some of the behavior, it does not have to be an excuse. It's completely appropriate for parents to have rules, consequences, and expectations for their child with epilepsy. In fact, structure, routine, and consistent expectations and consequences help all children learn to reg-ulate themselves. It's hard for parents sometimes because they feel bad for their child with epilepsy and what they have to go through, but in fact, behavioral dysregulation is a sign that a child needs more parenting and structure, not less.

Most persons who take ASMs to control their seizures do not experi-ence serious and intolerable side effects from them. In some cases, how-ever, the side effects from taking medication may affect an individual's behavior and/or emotional state. Such changes may include an impair-ment of motivation, mood, anger, aggression, alertness, or concentra-tion.

Autism Spectrum Disorder

Research shows an association between autism spectrum disorder (ASD) and seizures/epilepsy. Children with ASD are more likely to have seizures, and children with epilepsy are more likely to meet criteria for ASD. Diagnostic criteria for ASD have changed over the years, and it's now considered a spectrum from mild social communication difficul-ties to more substantial communication problems, repetitive behaviors, and restricted interests. Terms like *Asperger's syndrome* and *pervasive developmental disorder* (PDD) are now considered as falling under the umbrella of ASD. Children with ASD can also have a range of intellec-tual ability and level of functioning.

Current (*DSM-5*) criteria for ASD are (1) persistent deficits in social communication and social interaction across multiple contexts (such as lack of reciprocity, difficulty with nonverbal communication, difficulty forming relationships) and (2) restricted, repetitive patterns of behavior, interests, or activities (such as stereotyped movements, insistence on sameness, atypical sensory reactions, or restricted interests that are atypical in intensity or unusual in content). While many children have difficulties in both of these areas to some degree, the symptoms must also cause impairments in the child's life to warrant a diagnosis of ASD.

These are some stories we've heard, with examples of how to approach some of the comorbidities we've discussed.

Mrs. Christiansen brought us a letter from Billy's teacher. It said, "We have enjoyed having Billy in our kindergarten this year. He is a charming, adorable little boy. However, he did so poorly on his reading readiness test that we all feel he should spend another year in kindergarten. We would like you to come in for a meeting with us at your convenience." Mrs. Christiansen asked, "Should we tell her about Billy's epilepsy? He hasn't had a seizure since he started taking levetiracetam more than a year ago."

The first thing we would recommend is that she (along with other caregivers, if appropriate) meet with the teacher and find out more about Billy's problems in school. Have there been other problems, or did he just do poorly on the reading readiness test? Is he immature in other ways in school? How does his ability to learn games and other things compare to that of his peers? Does the teacher think that this is just a problem of maturity, which would be solved by repeating kindergarten, or are there other problems as well?

Teachers usually have a great deal of experience in identifying school problems, and the teacher's impressions can be of great help to you and to your child's physician in sorting out the problems and in finding the proper directions in which to proceed.

The second step would be to meet with the physician, to get advice about the teacher's impressions and suggestions. Do we all agree with the school? Is Billy one of the younger children in the class; might he benefit from another year there? Is he immature in other social ways? Does he act more like a 5-year-old than the usual 6-year-old who is starting first grade? Is he intellectually slower than normal? Is he a child with a specific learning problem? We often cannot answer these last two questions without psychological testing.

Does every child who is like Billy need testing? We would say no, but whether a child does or does not need testing will depend on the opinion of the teacher and on our assessment. We are often asked, "Is this neurological?" Our answer is always, "Yes. Learning problems are always neurological." Learning resides in the brain, not in the foot or heart. If a child isn't learning, it's because they can't or don't use their brain as expected. This does not mean that Billy has a neurological problem or that he needs to see a neurologist. It means that everyone (including the teacher) needs to assess the situation carefully and find the best educational strategy to manage it.

Those are the suggestions we would give to any parents who received that note from their child's teacher. The only thing different about Billy is that he has had seizures and is on levetiracetam. Yes, they should tell the teacher about Billy's seizures. They might also ask her if she has seen any daydreaming or other evidence that he may have been having subtle seizures in school. We would also be concerned about the possible role of the medication. With some medications, we would recommend checking a blood level to see if drug level is too high and possibly interfering with Billy's learning. We might also consider changing to another ASM (if Billy needed to continue medication) to see if his performance improved. There is no way to be absolutely certain that the medication is not interfering with learning and behavior except to take the child off that medicine and, if necessary, change to another medicine.

"This was the third time this fall that the teacher has called us in for a meeting. She says that Joshua is disruptive to the class. He bites, fights, and won't sit still. His reading is terrible, and she's afraid that he is going to be expelled. What should we do? Can they expel someone from the second grade? I think that the real problem is that the teacher is afraid that he'll have a seizure in class and really just wants him out."

We would begin to analyze this problem by asking the parents to tell us more about Joshua. What sort of a child is he? Is he having these types of behavioral problems at home? Are they new? When did they first start? Did he have similar problems last year in first grade? Was there anything particular that might have caused them? What was the relationship of the onset of these problems to the onset of his seizures and to the initiation of his antiseizure medication?

Behavioral problems such as biting and fighting can come from many different sources. Any of the antiseizure medications can cause behavioral changes such as this. If the change began shortly after the start of a new medication, then perhaps a different medication should be tried. Behavioral changes rarely occur weeks or months after the child has been on the same medicine, however, unless there has been a change in the dose. New behavioral problems can be caused by psychological disturbances initiated by problems at home or in school; they can be caused by the teacher's behavior toward the child and the child's reaction to his teacher's behavior. Does Joshua know about his seizures? Is he afraid or embarrassed by them? When people are anxious, they can get nasty or lash out at others. Perhaps a careful explanation of his seizures would alleviate some of his fears, and this might allow him to be less aggressive in school. It's also possible that he's acting out because he's frustrated about not being able to keep up with his classmates.

Discussing the problems and the parents' concerns with the teacher (or the principal) and with their child's physician can help them to sort through these different causes. Whatever the cause, the recent change in Joshua's behavior certainly is reason for concern and investigation. It is a common symptom of problems that require solutions. It could be Joshua's unconscious way of asking for help.

"Jasmine's grades are terrible. She's in high school, and this is such an important time for her future. She was a solid B student until her seizure, but since then she doesn't even finish her homework. Her last report card was Cs and Ds, and she now says that she wants to drop out of school and get a job. Could this be due to her medicine?"

In Jasmine's case, as in Joshua's, there are many potential sources for her problems. These could include romantic relationships, problems with friends, home problems, changes in school, insecurity about her future, depression, and concern and embarrassment over her seizures. These could all affect schoolwork and should be explored in talking with

Jasmine. We would check the blood level of her medication, and if it was high, lower the dose. If it wasn't, we would strongly consider changing to another medicine. While phenobarbital and phenytoin are the medications that most frequently affect learning, they are rarely used in children now, but such effects can follow use of any of the ASMs. Even as we were lowering or changing the medicine, we would explore with Jasmine what she knows about her seizures and her reaction to them. We would want to know how seizures have changed her lifestyle and her sense of self-esteem. We would ask about symptoms of depression and try to help her cope better with her epilepsy, whether or not this was the cause of her school problems. Perhaps she needs to talk with another teen who had similar problems with seizures. Or perhaps she needs even more support and counseling.

"Circe's teacher called us this week because she is daydreaming in class. We had told the teacher to watch for seizures, and now she thinks that Circe is having absence seizures again. Should we increase her medicine?"

Circe could be having more absence seizures. Perhaps this alert teacher has identified the problem early. Have the parents seen any at home? Is Circe aware of missing things during class? Is it possible that the teacher is just watching too closely and misinterpreting things? Perhaps we should first check the blood level to be certain that she is taking the medication and taking enough. Perhaps we should see Circe and hyperventilate her to see if we can produce one of her spells. If we can't be sure in the office, we might want to have another EEG, to see if she is still having many electrical episodes. In this way we can sort out if Circe has a problem and the best approach to correcting it.

CHAPTER 17

From Infancy to College

Navigating the Educational System

"Should I tell the school about my child's epilepsy?"

"How do I know what to ask for to support my child in school?"

Children and adolescents with epilepsy are at increased risk of academic underachievement, even when their seizures are well controlled. In fact, attention or learning problems are often identified prior to the first seizure and are thought to reflect the underlying brain condition. Academic underachievement is most likely multifactorial, resulting from the effects of neurological, neurocognitive, and psychosocial factors as well as the impact of other elements such as medication and missing a lot of school.

Remember:

• There is no reason to worry about the possibility of school problems if your child is not encountering and demonstrating problems.

• Most children with epilepsy do well in school.

• Most children with epilepsy do not have learning problems or social problems in school.

You should also remember that many children without epilepsy have problems of various kinds in school. Thus, even if your child does have problems in school, they may not be related to epilepsy itself. Learning problems, shyness, aggressive behavior, inattention, and reading problems are among the many school problems that can be related or unrelated to epilepsy.

If there are significant concerns about a child's school functioning, parents and teachers may decide the child needs extra help or support in school and may want to formalize services or accommodations to make sure the child has a successful academic experience. This chapter outlines the process of determining whether your child needs formal services and supports, and how to get them implemented through the public school system.

The Laws and Your Child's Rights

Several federal laws ensure that all children in the United States have access to a free and appropriate public education (FAPE). Despite the knowledge that children and adolescents with epilepsy are at risk for poor school performance, many do not receive services.

The three primary laws that apply to students with epilepsy are the Individuals with Disabilities Education Act, typically referred to as IDEA (2004), Section 504 of the Rehabilitation Act of 1973, often simply called Section 504 (1973), and the Americans with Disabilities Act, or ADA (1990).

Seizures and Epilepsy in School

Parents can certainly decide whether to inform the school if their child has a single seizure, has infrequent seizures, or has been diagnosed with epilepsy.

School health services can be an important part of the school team for a student with epilepsy, particularly if the child has frequent daytime seizures. Open communication between school health professionals, parents, and potentially the student's medical providers is advisable. School health professionals can provide training and information to the school team so that they can better understand the student's condition and be more comfortable in teaching them.

Models of school health services vary across the country. State nursing regulations mandate what care must be provided by registered nurses, licensed practical nurses, and health technicians and aides. It cannot be expected that there will be a full-time nurse in each school. Many school systems operate on a cluster model, where a registered nurse oversees several schools, and where each school may have a health technician.

These regulations may affect the school placement of the student with epilepsy who has a medical order for any medication administration, whether it is routine antiseizure medication or an emergency medication such as rectal diazepam (Diastat) or nasal midazolam (for older children) for a prolonged or recurring seizure. There may be occasions for a student with epilepsy to be placed in a school that is not their geographically assigned school, so they have access to proper nursing personnel. This would be considered acceptable if the peers and educational program are appropriate and there is no undue negative impact.

Home (and hospital) instruction is available to students who experience extended absences, usually several weeks, for health-related issues, but who are well enough to benefit from instruction. Some students with epilepsy experience intermittent absences, especially in periods when their seizures are not being well controlled on current medication and/or diet. Although not standard everywhere, more school systems are offering intermittent home teaching for students with chronic health conditions that cause these sporadic absences.

Seizure Action Plans

School health professionals are responsible to see that medication and diet orders are followed in the school setting during school hours. An emergency plan is also advisable, including when 911 would be accessed, when a parent should be called, and when a student should return to class, as well as a plan to have sufficient medication on hand for any emergency that might cause students to remain in the school building longer than usual. It is important that this plan be developed with the parent and school personnel together.

Special Education Eligibility

Children with disabilities from birth through 21 years of age may be eligible for special education services. IDEA outlines specific eligibility categories for special education, which include intellectual disability;

hearing impairments (including deafness); speech or language impairments; visual impairments (including blindness); serious emotional disturbance; physical or orthopedic impairments; autism; traumatic brain injury; multiple disabilities; other health impairments; or specific learning disabilities.

Epilepsy is not one of the "defined handicapping conditions"; if a student's epilepsy adversely affects their educational performance such that they need special education and related services, however, the student may be identified as a student in the category "other health impairment" as defined in IDEA.

Each student who qualifies for services has those services outlined in an individualized educational program (IEP). The basic components of an IEP include a description of the student's present academic functioning, including how the disability affects their progress in general education, measurable annual goals, and short-term objectives, as well as set intervals at which progress will be reviewed. The IEP must also include specifics of the types and amounts of special education and related services, any supplementary aids and services, a statement of any testing accommodations needed, a description of the location where services will be provided, and an explanation of the extent to which the student will be away from nondisabled peers.

A student with epilepsy who does not qualify for special education services under IDEA may receive support under Section 504 of the Rehabilitation Act of 1973. Section 504 is a civil rights law that protects persons with disabilities from discrimination related to their disabilities. It ensures that a student with a disability has "equal access" to an education. The student may receive accommodations and modifications as well as some services to ensure this equal access. Like IDEA, Section 504 applies to federally funded and federally conducted programs (e.g., public schools).

To be eligible for protections under Section 504, the student must have a "physical or mental impairment that substantially limits at least one major life activity." Major life activities include walking, seeing, hearing, speaking, breathing, learning, reading, writing, performing math calculations, working, caring for oneself, and performing manual tasks.

The General Process: Eligibility Determination, IEP/IFSP/504 Development, and Placement

The first step in the process is the referral. Anyone may refer a child for special education services, including the parent, the teacher, or an outside provider such as a pediatrician. This request should be in writing. The process begins with an interdisciplinary team meeting, including the parent, to review the referral and determine if there is evidence that the child may have a disability and need assessment. If so, the process proceeds with assessment to determine if there is a disability, defining the nature and extent of the disability, developing the IEP, determining services needed, and then review and reevaluation.

A child who has problems in school, whether or not they have epilepsy, should receive a careful evaluation to identify their strengths and weaknesses. Only then will the teachers be able to find the best way to help them learn. Evaluation for services under IDEA requires that the school review various measures that assess academic, developmental, and functional information. A single measure cannot be the only criterion for determining eligibility and designing an educational program. Often, schools require assessments from several disciplines to get a complete picture of the child's functioning.

Typically, schools will request a *psycho-educational* evaluation, which can be done by a school psychologist or outside provider. This consists of a psychological evaluation (e.g., an IQ test) and an educational evaluation (assessment of the child's level of academic abilities across reading, math, and writing). Sometimes the school will also request occupational therapy, physical therapy, speech and language, vision, or assistive technology evaluations. In children with neurological conditions, it may be helpful to get an outside neuropsychological evaluation to thoroughly assess brain-behavior relationships, including attention, learning, memory, language, executive functioning, visual-spatial skills, and other aspects of thinking and reasoning. Note that schools are required to consider evaluations done by other (not district-based) professionals, but do not have to accept the recommendations of those providers.

Through these evaluations, the school team will then make an "eligibility determination," deciding whether a child is eligible to receive services under IDEA. If a child is determined to be eligible, the school team, along with parents (and, if old enough, the child/teenager), will develop specific goals, services, proposed modifications to the curriculum, and suggested accommodations in an individualized education program (IEP) or individualized family services plan (IFSP). This document drives the placement. IDEA requires that a child's educational needs be met in the least restrictive environment. This could be regular classes with support within the classroom (*push in*), regular classes with some specialized classes (*pull out*), specialized classrooms, or in some cases specialized schools.

The processes for determining who is eligible for services under Section 504 are not specified within the legislation. Most school systems have set up their own processes, including a team that reviews information for eligibility. If the team feels special education or related services might be needed rather than or in addition to modifications and accommodations, the student must be evaluated. In either case, all information is gathered for review so that a 504 plan can be determined.

Although many students with epilepsy are eligible for services, modifications, or accommodations under Section 504, a student with epilepsy is not automatically covered by Section 504. If, for example, the student's seizures are under control with medication, there are no side effects from their medications, and their medications need not be administered in school, there may be no need for modifications or accommodations for equal access to a free appropriate education.

Early Intervention Services and IFSP

IDEA includes the Child Find mandate. Child Find requires all school districts to identify, locate, and evaluate all children with disabilities, regardless of the severity of their disabilities.

IDEA supports infants and toddlers with disabilities, and those who are at risk of developing disabilities, by mandating early intervention services. Early intervention services can include special education, physical, occupational, or speech/language therapies, nursing services, assistive technology, or case management. Children are eligible for early intervention services from birth to 3 years old.

Infants or toddlers with epilepsy might be eligible for services from an early intervention program if their seizures or underlying medical conditions interfere with their development and either cause them to have a developmental delay or to be at risk of having a disability. The services are recorded in a document called an individualized family services plan (IFSP), which has components similar to the IEP but with a focus not only on the needs of the child but also of the family and their part in facilitating development. Some children who receive early intervention services do not need further services when they turn 3; others transition into the special education system.

School Age: IEP vs. 504 Plan

Since the provisions of IDEA and Section 504 are the primary means of providing support to school-age students with epilepsy, it is important to understand more about the differences between the two.

Under Section 504, the mandate is to provide an education that is comparable to the education provided to students without disabilities. Students don't receive direct special education services under Section 504 but can receive related services and accommodations that are meant to provide access to general education.

The purpose of IDEA is different: "to ensure that all children with disabilities have available to them a free appropriate public education that emphasizes special education and related services designed to meet their unique needs and prepare them for further education, employment and independent living." IDEA is meant to design an individualized program and placement, whereas Section 504 provides support for a student to remain in a more typical placement with accommodations.

Any direct services, such as individualized instruction, small group instruction, occupational therapy, speech therapy, and physical therapy, would (usually) be provided through an IEP. It's important to note that to be provided through an IEP, these services must be "educationally relevant." As such, therapies through an IEP do not have the same goals as traditional outpatient therapies. For example, an occupational therapy evaluation through an IEP may focus on determining the best way for a child to produce work (e.g., writing vs. typing) but would not focus on things like strength and fine motor dexterity.

IDEA requires parental notice in writing on a specified timeline. Parents must be invited to attend meetings throughout all steps of the process for referral, assessment, identification, IEP development, review, and reevaluation. School systems must be able to show that they have informed parents of their rights at each meeting.

Section 504 requires that the school develop a plan but does not require a written document. Having a written plan, however, is helpful for parents and schools to verify what is expected, and to monitor whether the school is compliant in providing the services, modifications, or accommodations agreed on in the plan.

Any needed accommodations and modifications should be written into the student's IEP or 504 plan. While these terms are not defined by the laws, in general an accommodation allows the student to complete the same assignment or test as other students but with a change in the setting, format of presentation, response mode, or schedule. On the other hand, a modification is an adjustment to an assignment or test that changes what the assignment or test measures. IEPs are likely to include both accommodations and modifications, whereas many 504 plans typically include accommodations rather than modifications.

Transition Planning

For students over 16 years old who have IEPs, a transition plan must also be included. This transition plan should address goals for the eventual move from school services to functioning in higher education, employment, or independent living.

When a student graduates from high school or reaches the age of 22, entitlement to the provisions under IDEA end. IDEA does not extend to college or employment, whereas Section 504 provides protection in preschool, elementary and secondary school, postsecondary educational settings, employment, and community accessibility. Increasingly, students with disabilities plan to attend postsecondary schools, including two- and four-year colleges, as well as vocational, or career, schools. Most of these entities receive some type of public funding, and thus, compliance with Section 504 is extended to them.

Several of the requirements are different beyond high school. Postsecondary schools are required not to provide free appropriate public education but, rather, to provide appropriate academic accommodations to ensure that they do not discriminate based on disability. To receive the provisions of Section 504, students in the postsecondary setting must identify themselves as a student with a disability. The student is responsible for knowing and following the procedures the school has established to obtain adjustments afforded them by Section 504. When providing accommodations, the postsecondary school is not required to lower expectations or to effect substantial modifications to requirements. Students need to understand their needs and learn self-advocacy to be successful in obtaining the services they need.

CHAPTER 18

Playing, Sports Participation, and Other Activities

Participation in sports and other activities is an important part of the process of growing up. There are, of course, marked variations in individuals' athletic ability, developmental level, coordination, and interest in sports. Whether it's group play during recess, team sports like Little League, soccer, and lacrosse, or individual sports like swimming, karate, and riding, sports are important to a child's personal and social development. They offer an opportunity to participate with others, to share, and to learn teamwork and self-discipline, which are skills important to the development of personality, self-esteem, confidence, and character. While participation in organizations, such as Scouts, clubs, religious groups, and so on, can also be important to the development of self-esteem and character, children with epilepsy are less likely to be excluded from these organizations than they are from sports. We strongly believe no child should be deprived of the opportunities that these activities provide, and we advocate for inclusion to the fullest extent possible.

Q. *"Can I let my child go out and play?"*
A. Of course! You not only can but you should let them go out and play, go on trips, and sleep at a friend's house. "But suppose they have another seizure?" That's a risk you have to take. A careful analysis of risks is an important part of raising any child. It is a particularly important part of raising a child with the uncertainties of epilepsy. It is the crucial ingredient in avoiding overprotection. Their ability to run around and their

intelligence are the same as before the seizures. Most children with epilepsy are neither intellectually disabled nor learning disabled. For most such children, the only impairment is that, from time to time, they may experience a seizure.

Q. *"But don't they have a disability?"*
A. The answer is *no. They can still do what they were able to do before seizures began.* They can still run and play, go to school, sleep over at a friend's house. There is virtually *nothing* that a child who has had a few seizures cannot do. Obviously, all these decisions depend on how well the seizures are controlled. "Can he ride a bike?" Sure. The chances of having a seizure while riding his bike are very small, and if he is wearing a helmet, he is at only minimally greater risk than before the seizures. You may want to limit where he is riding. "Can she swim?" Absolutely, but swimming must be supervised, just as *every* child's swimming must be supervised. And it's wise to let the lifeguard know. "Isn't there a higher risk that she could drown or have a seizure in the water?" Yes, but only a *slightly* higher risk, since she has had only occasional seizures and may never have another one. Technically, your child may have a disability. They may fit the government definition that enables a person to obtain special services if the seizures interfere with education or work. But having a disability is very different from being disabled.

A handicap is often superimposed by society, parents, friends, or schools. People can also impose it on themselves.

Camps
Many of our children with epilepsy think that they are the only one in the world who is different, even if their classmates can't see the differences. They do not know anyone else with seizures. They have never even seen a seizure. Camps for children with epilepsy can often help develop a child's self-esteem. They will see that children with epilepsy are as different as their classmates. They will find that some children with seizures have many more disabilities than they do. They may also find that some children are brighter or more athletic than they are. They will find that they are just like all the other children in many ways, one of

them being that they all have seizures. Good self-esteem is the greatest gift you can give to your child, perhaps especially if they have seizures.

Many Epilepsy Foundation affiliates run summer camps for children with epilepsy. The camps are of varying length and expense. Some are only for the children with epilepsy. Others include siblings. Some are for children with multiple seizures; others also welcome those whose seizures are controlled or outgrown. Camps for children with epilepsy are often held at the same time as a camp for children without epilepsy. The inclusion of children with little or no handicap allows everyone to develop a realistic perspective on epilepsy and enables them to teach and become role models for one another.

While requiring more staffing and volunteers, these camps can be rewarding experiences for adolescents and adult volunteers. Siblings and parents might participate as counselors. The camps offer an opportunity to talk with other people who have epilepsy and often provide an opportunity for a child who has epilepsy to see for the first time what a seizure looks like to someone else.

If your Epilepsy Foundation affiliate does not have a camp, a group of parents might like to get one started. And the affiliate may be able to recommend a good camp that happily accepts children who have seizures and provides appropriate supervision.

On the other hand, finding a well-staffed inclusive camp that welcomes children with epilepsy can also be a wonderful experience and certainly mimics the wider world.

Q. *What do I write on all those school or camp forms now that she's had several seizures? Is she 'an epileptic'?"*
A. No, your child is not "an epileptic." They are a child who has had seizures. They are a child with epilepsy. First of all, they are a child, a person, an individual; they are not defined by the disorder. Most of the time they do not have seizures. Most of the time they are their normal selves. Seizures, or epilepsy, are a brief interlude in their life. But labeling is a big problem. The terms *epilepsy* and *epileptic* carry many myths and misconceptions. Unfortunately, the labels are often used in the pejorative sense. Labels are to be avoided unless they have some clear benefit

for your child. One expert has stated that a good reason not to treat after a first seizure (other than that it isn't of any benefit) is that having to take medication once or twice a day is a constant reminder that you are different. It is a reminder to the parents, and a reminder to the child. It is a label and cannot help but affect the child's self-esteem.

Q. *"I've heard that the local epilepsy association runs a camp just for children with epilepsy. Is that a good idea for Johnny? Wouldn't he be better off with normal kids?"*
A. See? You've slipped already. Kids with epilepsy are normal kids. They just have seizures in addition.

We find that the best approach to a child who has had several seizures, who has now been diagnosed as having epilepsy, is for you to gain a realistic acceptance of your child's limitations (if any) and to focus on their potential. This requires a conscious effort to put aside your anxiety and concern about all the things that could happen. This is not easy to do. It requires acceptance of the fact that there are risks inherent in rearing any child and that most children with epilepsy, especially those whose epilepsy is controlled, face only slightly greater risks than other children.

Children who have severe or difficult-to-control epilepsy and those who have additional impairments, such as intellectual disability, cerebral palsy, or learning disabilities, also require realistic acceptance. It is important that these children, too, be encouraged to reach their full potential and that additional disabilities not be superimposed (see Chapter 25).

Sports

Unfortunately, it is not realistic to make a single blanket statement about sports participation for all people with epilepsy. Decisions about participation must be based on an individual's circumstances, the type of seizures, and his or her degree of seizure control. The decision must, further, be based on the risks of the particular sport and the accommodations that can feasibly be made for that individual. The American Academy of Pediatrics does not consider free climbing, skydiving, hang gliding, or scuba diving to be safe.

The rules governing participation of children with epilepsy in sports should, in other words, be based on common sense. Each decision should be individualized. With that said, some more specific guidelines can be helpful in aiding families to make an informed decision.

Group Sports

Baseball, soccer, lacrosse—the list goes on. These sports are generally fine, and in fact, individuals with epilepsy can even be found on professional teams of these various different sports. With the proper protective equipment, these sports are usually encouraged. In terms of contact sports, the main concern is the chance of head or bodily injury, but children with epilepsy are not necessarily more likely to be hurt than other children. With that said, tackle football, rugby, and ice hockey have a higher incidence of injuries than most other sports, and participation in them should probably be limited to children with well-controlled seizures, as should wrestling, because children who have a seizure while participating may not be able to protect themselves from injury. Boxing should be avoided by all children because of the risk of head injuries.

Climbing

Any activity that involves heights should be undertaken only with harnesses and proper protective gear. This is true for children with and without epilepsy.

Swimming

No matter what, your child should always be closely supervised when in the water, and at least one person who is watching your child should (1) be familiar with CPR and (2) know that the child they are watching has epilepsy. Children with well-controlled seizures can swim competitively. If seizures are frequent or poorly controlled, children should be within arm's reach of a responsible adult and wear a lifejacket when in the water. Generally speaking, children with epilepsy should swim only in clear water; swimming in a lake, bay, or ocean is much more dangerous than swimming in a pool, as they can be difficult to locate if they slip under the water. Any child swimming in open water should wear a life jacket.

Gymnastics

Participation in gymnastics depends on the event. The closer your child is to the floor, the safer it is. Only children whose seizures are well controlled should consider performing on the high bar, uneven parallel bars, vaults, or rings. The parallel bars can be safer but still pose some risk depending on the exercise being performed. Floor routines and the pommel horse pose little risk.

Horseback Riding

Horseback riding is generally a safe activity, particularly for children with infrequent seizures. For children with frequent or poorly controlled seizures, a responsible adult should walk alongside the horse. Competitive horseback riding should be reserved only for children with well-controlled seizures.

Other Considerations

Q. *"Does my son need to wear a special helmet to protect his head when he's playing?"*

A. The brain of someone with epilepsy is not usually more sensitive or susceptible to injury than the brain of anyone else. In contact sports where headgear is required, that headgear should be sufficient for the child with epilepsy. Minor trauma to the head, which can occur in all these sports, is unlikely to precipitate a seizure at the time of the injury. A true traumatic brain injury (TBI), however, can sometimes aggravate seizures in a person with epilepsy.

Q. *"The doctor had him hyperventilate in the office. It didn't cause a seizure, but could running hard and being out of breath cause a seizure while he is playing?"*

A. No. Hyperventilation during exercise is balanced by changes in body chemistry and does not produce a seizure. In fact, breathing deeply and more rapidly by exercising or running is necessary to meet the body's demands for oxygen. We took care of one young woman who was so sensitive to hyperventilation that with only a few deep breaths, she would experience seizures. The result was so reproducible that she participated in demonstrations for medical students every time she came to clinic for her check-up. Yet she was a long-distance bicycle rider and never had a seizure while riding.

Q. *My daughter is a competitive swimmer. She feels that her antiseizure medication slows her down, and she tends to skip it on the days before her meets. I'm afraid that she will have a seizure. What should I tell her?"*
A. You should tell her that the medication is not likely to interfere with her performance but that a seizure will definitely interfere. You should make a contract with her that if she is mature enough to take training and swimming seriously, then she is also mature enough to manage her seizures and to take her medication reliably. If she feels that the medications are slowing her down, she should discuss this with her neurologist. Perhaps the dose can be lowered, or the medication changed. Perhaps the medication could even be discontinued if she has been seizure-free for a sufficient period. But your daughter should not do this on her own.

Q. *"We've just moved to a new town, and Kaden hasn't had a seizure in almost a year. Should he tell his coach that he has epilepsy?"*
A. Yes. That is the only way the coach can provide adequate supervision and be prepared if another seizure occurs. It is important that you and your child be honest with the coach, just as you expect the coach to be honest with you.

Q. *"Would you let an adolescent with epilepsy participate in a marathon or in one of those triathlons? Does the stress of these increase the chance of seizures?"*
A. In general, stress of this sort does not increase the chance of a seizure. The training for the event might provide a good test. We would allow them to try. If the training seemed to increase the frequency of seizures, they should probably not compete. They may be distressed if they have a seizure during training, but it will probably be less distressing than not being allowed to try.

Q. *"It sounds as if you allow children with epilepsy to do almost anything that they're capable of. Is that correct?"*

A. Yes. Sports are an excellent way for your child to develop skills and self-confidence. These skills will be useful in adult life, whether or not the seizures are cured or controlled. Children with epilepsy should not be made to feel different because of the overprotectiveness of others who fear they will have a seizure. Accommodations should be sensible without being overly restrictive.

We think a little common sense goes a long way. Much of our advice is centered on maintaining safety and can be applied to all children. If a child could be injured in a sport or activity, then all children involved, not just children with epilepsy, should have adequate protection to prevent or minimize an injury and adequate supervision to treat the injury if an accident occurs. If a child has just started having seizures or has just started on new medication, then more supervision should be provided until the seizures are controlled or the degree of seizure control is ascertained.

We are aware that we are far more permissive than many physicians. You, your child's physician, and your child will need to weigh both the risks and the benefits of participation in any sport and make the decision that is best for your child.

CHAPTER 19

Driving and Epilepsy

Few activities in our modern society are as essential as driving. The ability to drive enables freedom and independence and may be a condition for employment. Conversely, inability to drive a car is tied to lack of self-esteem, isolation, and depression. In a survey of adults with epilepsy, it was listed as the top concern, above medication side effects, mood problems, or social embarrassment. Even today, as self-driving cars are becoming a reality, we are still a long way off from when having a license will not be critical. It is no wonder that parents of children with epilepsy often ask, "Will my child be able to drive?"

Q. *"Is it safe? How do you know my child won't have a seizure while driving my car?"*
A. Driving is risky business for everyone; however, it is important to remember that while epilepsy does pose some risk, that risk is relatively small compared with other causes of crashes, like alcohol. In a study of fatal car crashes, only 0.2 percent are attributed to a seizure, compared with 30 percent for alcohol-related crashes. The same study showed that the majority of all car crashes involving drivers with epilepsy were caused by driver error, not seizures. Therefore, the decision about whether your child can safely drive is one that must be made together with your child's neurologist and should be focused on determining your child's maturity level and assessing their individual risk of having a seizure behind the wheel of a car. It is also determined by state driving laws.

The first and best way to determine risk is the *seizure-free interval*, or the length of time a person has been seizure-free. In short, the longer a person has been seizure-free, the less likely they are to have a seizure, particularly while driving. Every state has their own laws governing how long a person must be seizure-free before obtaining (or reinstating) a driver's license, but these intervals generally range anywhere from 3 to 12 months. (Keep in mind, these laws also apply to learner's permits.) A 3-month seizure-free interval was proposed by the consensus statement from the American Academy of Neurology (AAN), American Epilepsy Society (AES), and the Epilepsy Foundation (EF). We also believe that this is a reasonable seizure-free interval.

Other factors may be considered, such as when seizures typically occur or whether awareness is preserved during the seizures. For example, if a person's seizures occur only while sleeping or if a person has seizures that are purely sensory while awake, that person may be permitted to drive, even if the seizures are not fully controlled. To be reasonable and sensible, we recommend that licensing procedures be guided by the type of seizure the individual has. Conversely, if a person has a history of medication noncompliance, particularly if they caused an accident as a result of a seizure in the past, that person may be required to be seizure-free for a longer period or may not be permitted to obtain a driver's license at all.

The chances of having a seizure while driving will obviously be determined in part by the amount of time the person spends at the wheel. That risk is also affected by fatigue, lack of sleep, alcohol, medication noncompliance or forgetting to take seizure medication, use of other medications, and many unknown factors. All these risk factors must be discussed prior to a person being cleared to drive.

Q. *"Can't we just keep the diagnosis to ourselves? Do we really have to report it?"*
A. Some families, when faced with the prospect of dealing with the paperwork and bureaucracy of their local motor vehicle administration, question whether they must really report their child's epilepsy diagnosis; we assure them that if their child wishes to drive, then it is nonnegotiable. Self-reporting for individuals with seizures is mandatory in all 50

states. Failure to follow regulations is not only illegal but may result in accidents. Accidents occurring when the driver's epilepsy is unreported, even if the accident is unrelated to a seizure, can result in problems with insurance coverage. Furthermore, it may prevent or delay an individual from getting a driver's license in the future.

Q. *"Doesn't my child's doctor report her to the state anyway?"*
A. Currently only six states require the physician to report the name of an individual who has had seizures; however, when a physician feels that an individual presents a "substantial risk to others" because the person is driving against medical advice, reporting may be necessary. It is important to keep in mind that you and your child's neurologist are a team. The goal is not to punish your child for having epilepsy but to help maximize your child's level of seizure control and keep everyone (including your child) as safe as possible. Reporting every seizure to your child's neurologist is critical and will enable your child's neurologist to make the necessary medication changes to allow your child to drive safely.

Q. *"What if my child's neurologist recommends weaning medication? My child doesn't want to stop driving."*
A. Most states do not have any specific rules or restrictions on driving following the weaning or discontinuation of ASMs. Nonetheless, patients and families should be aware of the risk of seizure recurrence when medication is reduced or stopped. In one study of individuals with epilepsy who had been in remission for 2 years, seizure recurrence was followed for a year after discontinuation of their medication. Overall, the rate of recurrence within 12 months was 30 percent. For those patients who were seizure-free 3 months after stopping their medication, however, their chance at being seizure-free at a year was 85 percent; for those who were seizure-free at 6 months, the likelihood of seizure freedom at a year was 91 percent. As you can see, the odds improved significantly the longer the person was seizure-free off medication. Therefore, your child's neurologist may ask that they stop or cut down on driving temporarily after medication changes to reduce the likelihood of a seizure happening while driving. We generally recommend that patients

refrain from driving for 3 months after ASMs are discontinued. Your state may also require the driver to report any change in medication. We find that the teenage driver is the big decision maker in these situations—don't be surprised if, faced with this situation, they say, "I need to drive and can't risk either losing my license or even taking 3 months off—don't touch my medications!"

Q. *"Every state is different, and information is always changing. Where can I get more information?"*
A. Standards change and recommendations evolve over time. Regularly updated information is available from local state authorities. You can also check out the "State Driving Laws Database" at the Epilepsy Foundation website for more information: https://www.epilepsy.com /driving-laws. In addition, your child's neurologist can reach out to the local MVA/DMV (they often know which neurologists and physicians are on the board) and ask questions on your behalf.

CHAPTER 20

Devices, Apps, and Websites

This chapter provides an overview of some modern devices, applications, and websites that might be helpful to families. It is by no means comprehensive and is not meant to endorse one product over another. Families should use it as a guide to what they might be looking for that would possibly be helpful to their individual circumstances.

Devices

People with epilepsy and their families have used various devices to try to improve care for many years. They include such simple things as a MedicAlert bracelet and more advanced computerized electronic items such as watches.

MedicAlert bracelet (https://www.medicalert.org/medicalert-medical -ids). The bracelet or necklace helps providers understand your medical issues with a unique Member ID number that can be used to share your Emergency Health Record with providers. It also provides basic information such as that the individual has epilepsy. It comes in a wide variety of styles that are even appropriate for children.

Helmets. Many manufacturers make helmets that can protect your child's head from injury, and some even come with face guards. Although helmets don't prevent all concussions (as any football player knows), they do provide some protection against more severe trauma, and the American Academy of Pediatrics certainly advocates their use for children riding bicycles.

Medication reminders. A wide variety of devices try to improve medication adherence. These include simple pillboxes with the day and time of day on them to serve as organizational aides and passive reminders. There are also more sophisticated devices with alarm timers that will alert you or your child to take the medication. This type of device can enhance your child's independence and provides a quick check at the end of the day that all the appropriate medication has been given. Two are listed on the Epilepsy Foundation (EF) site: e-pill (www.epill.com) and TabTime (www.tabtime.com).

Seizure alarms and alert devices. EF provides a thoughtful guide, "Considering a Seizure Alert Device" (https://www.epilepsy.com/sites /core/files/atoms/files/DAS100_Seizure_Alert_Devices_09-2018 _FINAL2.pdf), which examines what your goals are, your living situation, device portability, cost, and how the information obtained by the device will be shared.

As clinicians, we are aware that one major concern is what are called *false positives.* The device alerts you and your child when all that's happened is movement, perhaps in the restless period when a child is falling asleep. These false alarms can be very disruptive to you and your child. We also know that they are not 100 percent accurate, especially if a child has multiple types of seizures. And we do not have any evidence that they can prevent sudden unexpected death in epilepsy (SUDEP). They may, however, allow you to provide help sooner than you might have been able to do without them.

The earliest form of alert device was a mattress device. These detect unusual motion, typically fast or jerking movements. Some also include cameras and can produce either a sound alarm or use a pager. Others detect sound. Still others measure actual muscle contraction through changes in the skin. And more recently, a number of wearable devices (watches and applications to be uploaded to them) have been developed. In addition to the device purchase price, many require monthly subscriptions so that caretakers can be notified. One is called the Embrace 2 and is cleared by the FDA (https://www.empatica.com/embrace2/). Our colleagues at Johns Hopkins have also developed an app for the Apple Watch called EpiWatch, which is part of ongoing research to improve detection and prediction. These devices not only detect but send out predetermined notifications to obtain help. As we've learned more about better ways of detecting seizures, often by evaluating devices within epilepsy monitoring units, we've learned that many parameters that can lead to improved systems and hopefully fewer false positives and false negatives, when actual seizures are missed. In an excellent review funded by the Epilepsy Foundation (*Epilepsia* 2020;61(S1):S11–S24), the authors are optimistic that these devices will improve in the future. Devices will likely be designed to be multimodal, able to measure more than one biological parameter, as the EpiWatch does. In fact, many researchers are working on devices that will reliably predict a seizure so that it could potentially be prevented. It's beyond the scope of this book to individually list all these devices, but they are readily found on the internet. Many require prescriptions from a physician, which is quite appropriate, since you should discuss whether a particular device might be helpful for your child.

Apps

Apps vary widely, as could be expected. The major types are seizure tracking (diaries), health care sites that also keep records of medications and side effects, information resources, and notification systems. We list a few to provide a sense of the scope, but clearly this is not meant to be comprehensive. Again, please check with your child's health care provider for their opinion on sites that you find or use so that they are kept well informed of the efforts you are taking to care for your child.

App Examples

Seizure tracking: Seizure Tracker, Simple Seizure Diary, Seizario, Epilepsy Journal

Health care management: MyChildren's, My Seizure Diary, EpiDiary, Epsy

Information resources: Seizure First Aid

Notification systems: Snug Safety, Aura: Seizure Helper, SeizAlarm: Seizure Detection

Websites

Throughout the book we mention websites that are particularly relevant to the subject matter being discussed. In fact, one of the biggest problems, as well as the largest blessing, is how much information is available today for parents and people with epilepsy. As is true for most subject matter, the real problem is sorting out the reliable and helpful from the misleading. We've advocated throughout this book that you should use your health care provider and their team as an important filter and source of advice. Certainly, a primary resource should be the Epilepsy Foundation (https://www.epilepsy.com). This site is carefully organized by professionals who have devoted their lives to the service of people with epilepsy, and it is carefully curated by a professional advisory board that oversees updating it with reliable information. Here are some other important resources, which we've listed in alphabetical order.

American Epilepsy Society (https://www.aesnet.org). This is a professional society that includes physicians, surgeons, nurses, social workers, psychologists, and others who are involved in research, care, and improving outcomes for people with epilepsy.

Center for Parent Information and Resources (https://www.parent centerhub.org). This is a source that supports parents who have children with disabilities. Very extensive.

Centers for Disease Control and Prevention: Disability and Health Information for People with Disabilities (https://www.cdc.gov /ncbddd/disabilityandhealth/people.html). Major clearinghouse for available resources.

Cure Epilepsy (https://www.cureepilepsy.org/). This site was founded by a group of parents who are dedicated to finding answers to help their children. They are a source for current information about a wide variety of topics, especially research and education.

International League Against Epilepsy (https://www.ilae.org). ILAE is a worldwide organization offering a wide variety of resources to professionals as well as patients. It is helpful in understanding epilepsy activity in your part of the world.

National Association of Epilepsy Centers (https://www.naec -epilepsy.org/). This is an organization of centers that provide various levels of epilepsy care. You can go there to find local and regional centers near you.

National Institute of Neurological Disorders and Stroke: Epilepsy Information Page (https://www.ninds.nih.gov/Disorders/All -Disorders/Epilepsy-Information-Page). The NINDS hosts a major site that provides an entry into information about treatment, research, clinical trials, organizations, and publications.

SUDEP Action (https://sudep.org/). This is a UK website devoted to raising awareness and promoting research and education about SUDEP.

If your child has been diagnosed with a specific syndrome or has undergone certain therapies, there is likely a parent group that will be helpful. For instance:

Charlie Foundation for Ketogenic Therapies (https://charliefoundation.org/)

Dravet Syndrome Foundation (https://www.dravetfoundation.org/what-is-dravet-syndrome/)

The Hemispherectomy Foundation (https://hemifoundation.homestead.com/welcome.html)

Lennox-Gastaut Syndrome (LGS) Foundation (https://www.lgsfoundation.org/)

National Organization for Rare Disorders: Rasmussen Encephalitis (https://rarediseases.org/rare-diseases/rasmussen-encephalitis/)

Tuberous Sclerosis Association (https://tuberous-sclerosis.org/)

CHAPTER 21

Insurance and Other Financial Issues

We could fill a book with discussion of insurance issues and some of the horror stories we have heard from patients. Therefore, we think it is important to pass on some tips we have collected over the years.

If you are about to change insurance companies, or you are trying to have your child covered, you should do careful research before signing on with any insurance company or insurance plan. We recognize that you may not have any choice about the coverage, but you should try to optimize the benefit to your child. Find out about the following issues.

• Will the company allow you to go to the doctor and hospital of your choice?

• Ask if your doctor and hospital are in or out of the company's network and find out what your proportion of financial responsibility (coinsurance) or copay will be.

• Is there an out-of-pocket maximum for you, and will the insurance company then cover 100 percent of the medical costs? Often insurance companies will tell you that they pay 100 percent, but that is 100 percent of what they consider to be reasonable and customary. That can be misleading, and you can wind up with out-of-pocket expenses that you did not anticipate. For example, if a hospital charges $1,200 per day and your insurance company says the reasonable and customary charge is $800 per day, that leaves you with $400 per day out of pocket, which can add up quickly if your child is hospitalized for any length of time.

Check the formulary to be sure that your child's medication will be covered. If your child's seizures are poorly controlled, ask your doctor what other medications they might try in the near future and be sure they're also on the formulary.

Before signing on with an insurance company, get in writing any "promises" that the company makes to you, such as "You can see any doctor you choose," or "You may go out of state to any hospital you would like."

We recommend that you talk to the financial offices of your child's doctor or hospital to find out which insurances they accept and which ones they bill directly, or whether you must pay out of pocket and then be reimbursed from your insurance. Paying out of pocket is prohibitive for most families, especially for ongoing treatment.

If your child qualifies for Medicaid in your state, consider carefully before you drop them from your insurance, because most hospitals do not accept Medicaid or State Children's Health Insurance Program (SCHIP) from a state other than their own, and you may want to use the services of a doctor or epilepsy center out of state. In addition, some physicians do not accept Medicaid.

The same premise holds true for children who go off to college and qualify for student insurance. They are only insured while actively enrolled, so if a child goes into the hospital for surgery and has to miss a chunk of time from school, they may not be covered. Since children can now be kept on parents' plans until they're 26 years old, many experts will tell you that it is best to carry children on your policy even if there is other coverage for them. Better overinsured than underinsured. In the past, people with epilepsy often had difficulty obtaining insurance because they had a preexisting condition. Currently that is no longer a problem.

Often you can enlist your primary care physician to help you get an appointment at an epilepsy center and to have it covered by insurance, by emphasizing that they are *specialists* in this area. Sometimes it is worth the financial investment, however it is paid, to go to an epilepsy center for a second opinion and then take those recommendations back to the physician who is caring for your child. Most physicians do not object to their patients' getting a second opinion.

If (or, unfortunately, more often when) coverage for epilepsy evaluation or treatment is denied, appeal! Insurance companies do not advertise their appeal process, but all companies have one. Decisions are sometimes overturned on appeal, especially if a physician or nurse calls and speaks to the insurance medical director. In insurance, as in life, the squeaky wheel gets the grease. It is also important to recognize, however, that many new antiseizure medications today are *very* expensive as a result of the pharmaceutical company's decision when they were first released. In those cases, the insurance companies are even more opposed to paying unless children fit very specific criteria for these drugs based on FDA approvals.

You should not have to go into financial debt to get good care for your child. That generally is not necessary. Many excellent physicians around the country are able to provide care for a child with epilepsy, and you should not feel that you have to move, mortgage your home, or take some other drastic measure to ensure that your child's epilepsy is adequately treated.

Another area of concern should be estate planning, particularly if you have a very disabled child. It is never too early to think about setting up the proper financial arrangements to be put in place once you and your partner can no longer care for your child, or after your death. No one will be here forever, and you cannot, nor should you, assume that your other children will take on the role of caretaker after you are gone. You should find a lawyer who is familiar with estate planning, who can advise you on the options that you have and how to put them in place. If you make these arrangements early on, you will feel relieved that your child will be taken care of. Your other children will be able to breathe easier as well. It is wonderful for siblings to take an active part in their brother's or sister's life, but they are not the parent. It is amazing how quickly time passes. Your child will be an adult before you know it. Your time together will be more enjoyable for you both if you know that you have done what you can to plan for their future.

CHAPTER 22

The Future

Epilepsy Care, Marriage, Pregnancy, and Children

Transition of Epilepsy Care

Although many children outgrow their epilepsy prior to reaching adulthood, the issue of transfer or transition of care to an adult setting must be addressed for many families. There is considerable difference between the family-centered care seen in pediatrics and the more typical patient-centered care for adults. If it appears that epilepsy may be an ongoing issue beyond the typical pediatric age range, a discussion of transition to adult care should happen sooner rather than later, perhaps even when your child is 12–13 years of age. Certainly, by the midteens, a discussion should occur about the best way to ensure optimal future care, perhaps in an adult epilepsy clinic that might be associated with the pediatric clinic, or with a single practitioner. This transition can often be done more smoothly when the practitioners can discuss the patient with each other, not simply by reading the patient's records. Typically, by 18 years of age (or perhaps after the first year of college to minimize the abrupt changes in a person's life), this process can be accomplished.

Marriage and Parenthood

Parents understandably wonder and worry about what their child's future holds for them and often hope that marriage and children will be part of it. Sadly, not so long ago, marriage of persons with epilepsy was prohibited by law in many states. The eugenics movement, relying on a US Supreme Court decision that supported not passing down impairing conditions to the next generation, was able to implement these laws. Fortunately, the rationale behind these laws was proved to be erroneous, and the laws were abolished. People who have a known genetic cause for their epilepsy should speak with appropriate counselors if they decide to have children. It should not prevent them from forming partnerships or marrying.

Q. *"Can I get married?"*
A. Of course! If a person with epilepsy is competent to be a spouse, however that competence is defined, there is no reason they should not get married. That is, if they want to get married, of course!

Q. *"Can I have children?"*
Q. *"Would pregnancy make my seizures worse?"*
A. Most women with epilepsy can bear children. There are some increased risks, however, some of which can be minimized if you work with your doctor before becoming pregnant. For instance, overall, birth defects occur in 4–6 percent of infants born to women who are being treated for epilepsy (twice the rate for the general population). But these risks are dependent on which medications are being used.

If you have questions about what might have caused your epilepsy in the first place or about the effect of pregnancy on other health problems, you should check with your physician before you decide to become pregnant.

Your seizures may change during pregnancy. Therefore, your obstetrician needs to know about your epilepsy, and your neurologist, about your plans to become pregnant. In about one-third of pregnant women, seizures get worse; in one-third, they improve; and in one-third, they are unchanged. Since we cannot predict which group you will fall into, your pregnancy should be monitored carefully. Pregnancy often affects blood levels of your epilepsy medications, so these levels will also need to be closely monitored.

Q. *"Can a person with epilepsy be a competent parent?"*
A. The answer is clearly yes! Most people who have epilepsy are extremely competent parents, just as we hope would be true for most

people without epilepsy. Individuals with epilepsy have personal strengths and weaknesses, just as others do. You will have to ask yourself and your partner whether you as individuals have the ability, maturity, and judgment to be good parents.

Sometimes people you trust can be helpful to you in thinking about these issues. That is for you to decide, but a "no" decision should not be based simply on the fact that you have epilepsy.

Q. *"Can someone who still has seizures be a good parent?"*
A. Absolutely, although the problems of being a parent with ongoing seizures may be more difficult, depending on the frequency of your seizures, their type, and even the time of day they occur. If your seizures are frequent and result in sudden loss of consciousness, you might drop or injure your child during a seizure. You may have to arrange for special help in the home or for childcare outside the home. But even so, you can be a good parent.

Risks of Pregnancy while Taking Antiseizure Drugs

Q. *"Should my epilepsy medication be reduced while I'm pregnant?"*
A. Pregnancy, especially early pregnancy, is not a good time to be changing antiseizure medications or to be adjusting them. Therefore, it is best to have a conversation with your physician to discuss treatment options *before* you plan to become pregnant. Some medications are more likely to affect the fetus than others. Some women may no longer need to be on several medications, and some may not need any medication at all. Whenever possible, the woman should be on the least number of medications, on the lowest dose, before becoming pregnant.

Since blood levels change during pregnancy, your medication levels should be monitored closely. We generally recommend that these levels be measured before you become pregnant and at least monthly starting in the second trimester. It is not uncommon for your neurologist to need to adjust the dosage based on changing blood levels as your pregnancy progresses.

Seizures increase during pregnancy in almost one of three women with epilepsy for four principal reasons. The first is that pregnant women are naturally fearful that taking drugs may affect the fetus, and therefore, they may fail to take their seizure medications according to schedule. A second reason is lack of sleep during pregnancy, which lowers the seizure threshold. A third cause of seizures during pregnancy is changes in the body's metabolism of drugs. Although such changes can cause blood levels to rise and thus cause toxicity, blood levels can also decline, leading to seizures. Your physician should closely follow your blood levels and provide appropriate adjustments. A fourth reason is hormones. Increased estrogen can increase seizures, while progesterone can decrease seizures. The balance of these hormones can shift a great deal during pregnancy.

Although there is little evidence that brief seizures injure the fetus, a prolonged seizure might affect your fetus, and any seizures might cause injury to you. Therefore, we strongly urge that pregnant women with epilepsy who need medication for seizure control continue to take the drug that has been controlling their seizures.

Q. *"Are there risks to my baby when I am taking antiseizure medications?"*
A. Yes, if a pregnant woman is on ASMs, there are risks to the baby. Those risks vary with the drug and are usually small.

No pregnant woman should be on antiseizure medication if it is not needed, and a woman who no longer needs medication should have it discontinued before she becomes pregnant. This must be done under a physician's supervision. And every pregnant woman should be on folate prior to becoming pregnant and should remain on it throughout pregnancy.

Every pregnancy, with epilepsy or without, carries some risk of a birth defect or developmental problem, of having a baby with some problems. Approximately 2 to 3 percent of all children will be born with some developmental abnormality. When a woman has, or has previously had, epilepsy but is not taking medication during the pregnancy, the risk of a child with an abnormality is minimally increased over the general population. We don't know why this is true, but it may be related to some as yet unknown genetic abnormality. Thus, this woman (no current seizures and no medications) has about a 95 percent chance of having a normal infant. If she is on medication, then the risk must be examined on an individual basis depending on data we have about each specific medication. The chance of having a child with congenital or developmental abnormalities is also increased if the father has or has had epilepsy, although the risk is lower than when the mother has it.

Each medicine poses different potential risks to the fetus; some are more serious than others, and some are more likely to cause problems.

Abnormalities vary with antiseizure medication and may be severe—such as spina bifida, congenital heart disease, or cleft palate—or minor, as in the length of the fingers.

Valproate (Depakote/Depakene)

Exposure to valproate/valproic acid in utero is associated with both major and minor abnormalities, including effects on the heart, bones, neurological system, and urogenital systems. It can also be associated with fetal valproate syndrome, which can cause craniofacial abnormalities, neural tube defects, skeletal anomalies, and cognitive problems. The benefits of continuing valproate during pregnancy should be weighed carefully against the risks, and the lowest dose should always be prescribed, as the risk of birth defects is decreased at lower doses. With that said, it is possible, and even likely, to have a healthy baby while taking valproate if switching to another medication is not a reasonable option.

Phenytoin (Dilantin)

This drug is believed by most people to carry an increased risk of cleft lip and palate, as well as of congenital heart disease. The risk of these problems is about 5 percent. Since these malformations occur during the first weeks of pregnancy, they cannot be prevented by stopping the drug after you realize you are pregnant. There is an increased risk of *fetal hydantoin syndrome* when the mother has been taking phenytoin. In this syndrome, the infant has blunted fingers and toes and small fingernails, is of slightly short stature, and has a small head. Whether such children are intellectually disabled remains a matter of debate. Some people feel that the risk of this syndrome is perhaps 20 to 30 percent. Others feel that the significance of these minor abnormalities is greatly overstated. Similar features may be found in children of a mother with epilepsy who has taken phenobarbital (fetal barbiturate syndrome) or one who has not been on medication at all.

Fetal hydantoin syndrome may be caused by the way certain women metabolize the drug. If you have had a baby who has the syndrome, your chances of having another affected child may be very high if you continue taking phenytoin (Dilantin) during your second pregnancy.

Other Antiseizure Medications

Phenobarbital and carbamazepine (Tegretol) may cause problems with the fetus that resemble hydantoin syndrome. The risks for both drugs appear to be slightly less than for phenytoin. Lamotrigine (Lamictal) can increase the risk of neural tube defects (spina bifida) if supplemental folic acid is not taken along with it prior to and during pregnancy. The risks to the fetus of newer anticonvulsant medications remain to be determined but are actively being studied, and we are learning more all the time. Levetiracetam (Keppra) and zonisamide (Zonegran) have been shown to be two of the safer antiseizure medications in pregnancy.

All women should be taking at least 800 mcg of folic acid a day if they are intending to get pregnant (or if they may become pregnant) and while they are pregnant. Your doctor may recommend a higher dose depending on the particular ASM you are taking.

Emily was 31 and desperately wanted to have a child. She had recently been placed on carbamazepine (Tegretol) because of a single seizure. She had a dilemma. Should she get pregnant with the risks of medication to the fetus, or should she stop the medication with the risks of a seizure to herself and the fetus? Although she realized that the risks of carbamazepine to her baby were relatively small, she could not accept the guilt of potentially causing a problem. She was worried about the possibility of spina bifida. She was also fearful of having a seizure while she was pregnant and of possibly injuring the baby. She was much less concerned about the potential effects of a seizure on her own active life.

We suggested a way out of her dilemma. Since she had had only a single seizure, the chances of her having another seizure were approximately 30 percent. If her medication was slowly discontinued, she could wait 3 to 6 months and see if another seizure occurred. She'd also have to stop driving for that period. After that time, the risk of recurrence would be even smaller, and she could become pregnant with greater security. If she had another seizure, then she would know that she needed an antiseizure medication and might try one with less potential risk to the fetus. Another possibility would be to substitute another medication, perhaps levetiracetam (Keppra).

Breastfeeding and Birth Control

Q. *"Can I breastfeed my baby?"*
A. Yes. While all the ASMs will appear in the mother's breast milk, they are usually in such low concentrations that they do not affect the baby. If you are taking phenobarbital or phenytoin and the baby becomes too sleepy, however, then the baby's blood level should be checked. If the level is too high, breastfeeding might be stopped for a few days.

Q. *"What about birth control?"*
A. Some ASMs increase the metabolism of birth control hormones and make them less effective. Therefore, if you are using birth control pills, particularly the mini-pill, and are taking certain ASMs, you might have a higher chance of becoming pregnant. Conversely, birth control pills can decrease the efficacy of some antiseizure medications like lamotrigine, meaning that you may need a higher dose of your seizure medication to control your seizures. You should always discuss the effects of your birth control pills on your ASM with your neurologist, and the effects of the ASM on the effectiveness of your birth control pills with your gynecologist.

Q. *"Since I have seizures, are there any risks of my child developing epilepsy?"*
A. Yes, there is a small risk of your children developing epilepsy. The risk of epilepsy in the child whose mother or father has epilepsy is about twice as great as when neither of the parents has epilepsy but is still relatively small. The risk of anybody's child having epilepsy is 1 to 2 percent.

If you or the child's father has epilepsy, your child has a 3 to 4 percent chance of having epilepsy. In addition, if you or your partner have a known genetic cause for your epilepsy, these risks might be somewhat different and need to be addressed with a genetic counselor.

Q. *"If I have children, will they be normal?"*
A. No one can give you a warranty on your child. Some abnormalities are not detectable even by our most sophisticated prenatal and intra-uterine screening. Some major problems are acquired at birth or are a consequence of later infection or trauma. Some genetic diseases cause epilepsy. Some risks are associated with antiseizure medications. There are some risks if you have previously had epilepsy.

If you are unwilling to take any risk, then you should probably not have a child. If you are willing to take some risk, then you, as well as most people with epilepsy, can have healthy children, unless you or your partner has epilepsy caused by certain specific genetic diseases, such as tuberous sclerosis or another metabolic condition that has a high like-lihood of being passed down genetically. If no cause has been found for your epilepsy or it is suspected to be genetic, you may want to con-sider genetic testing prior to becoming pregnant. This could help you determine if there is an underlying genetic cause for your epilepsy (e.g., a mutation in a specific gene that is known to cause seizures) and the likelihood of you passing it down to your offspring. If you'd like more information about genetic testing, talk to your neurologist to determine if genetic testing is appropriate. For more information on epilepsy and genetic testing, see Chapter 9. You should also speak with your child's physician about the possible risks associated with the ASM your child is taking.

Employment
Parents often worry that their child's epilepsy will affect or otherwise limit potential job opportunities when their child reaches adulthood. We'll start with the good news: right now, people with epilepsy are doing just about every job imaginable. They are physicians, nurses, lawyers, plumbers, electricians, IT specialists, entrepreneurs, writers, engineers,

professional athletes, artists, musicians—the list goes on. It's important to note that the mere existence of a preexisting epilepsy diagnosis does not necessarily exclude a person from certain jobs, contrary to popular belief. This may be particularly true if a person has been seizure-free and off medication for many years. Historically, people diagnosed with epilepsy were not allowed to serve in the US military, work as an airline pilot, bus driver, or commercial truck driver, or be employed as a law enforcement officer (in some states). Because these regulations change over time, individuals should check with the appropriate authorities regarding any restrictions.

This means that the overwhelming majority of jobs are fine for people with epilepsy. The ADA (Americans with Disabilities Act) specifically prohibits discrimination against qualified people with disabilities, including people with epilepsy, in employment. This means that employers can't exclude someone with a disability from any employment opportunity unless they are actually unable to perform the job. People with disabilities are also legally entitled to "reasonable accommodations," meaning employers are obligated to change the work environment or the way tasks are customarily performed to enable a person with a disability to experience equal employment opportunities, unless the accommodation imposes "undue hardship" on the employer (e.g., it is too expensive to implement, etc.). The Equal Employment Opportunity Commission (EEOC) also expanded its definition of epilepsy as a disability to include "limitations that occur as the result of seizures or because of side effects or complications that can result from medications used to control the condition," so protections and accommodations are not just for those who are having seizures in the workplace; they are for all people with epilepsy who need them.

With that said, individuals with epilepsy can have higher rates of unemployment, which is highly correlated with level of seizure control; individuals with intractable seizures are far more likely to be unemployed than those with well-controlled seizures. There are various reasons for this that may extend beyond the seizures themselves. For example, it is not uncommon for those with uncontrolled seizures to have higher levels of comorbid mental health conditions, such as anxiety or depression, or cognitive or motor impairments associated with their epilepsy. Individuals with epilepsy who are unable to work, or who are unable to work full time, can apply for federal disability benefits through the Social Security Administration. The process can be lengthy, and the criteria to qualify can be complex. If you need help with this process, you should reach out to your child's physician and your local Epilepsy Foundation chapter.

While the future can seem daunting after your child has been diagnosed with epilepsy, your child's future holds so much potential. With a few adjustments along the way, your child's dreams are still possible, whatever they may be.

PART V

Emotional AND Psychological Issues

CHAPTER 23

Initial Strategies and Overview

There are many different kinds of seizures, and each may affect you and your child in a different fashion. Some children will have only one seizure. Others may have many. You, the parent, will have to find a way of coping, and so will your child. The child's strategy will vary with age, and the strategies of all of you will vary with your personalities as well as with the type and frequency of seizures. But common themes run through all these variations.

The First Seizure

What You Should Know

"Ricky had a seizure!" his mother shouted to her husband over the phone. "He's on his way to the emergency room in an ambulance. They said that he had a grand mal seizure. Meet me there right away!"

A generalized tonic-clonic, "shaking" seizure (once called grand mal) is the type most frightening to parents. This one seizure has changed your life. Can you ever look at your child the same way again? Can you really let them go out and play in the backyard without watching them? Suppose they have another seizure? Maybe they could hurt themselves. What would the neighbors think if they knew? Will your best friend still let her son come over to play? Will she take the responsibility of watching them? How about the school? Do you want them to know? Do you want it on their records? Will the school allow your child to be normal, to do all the things their classmates are doing?

The first thing you need is information. You need to talk to your doctor about what they think caused the seizure, about tests and treatment, and about your child's future. In the case of a *provoked seizure*, when your child recovers and whatever caused the seizure is gone, the seizures will be gone. If the seizure was caused by a fever (a febrile seizure), your child will probably need a few tests but no long-term treatment and should outgrow these seizures as they get older. If the seizure was *unprovoked*, meaning there was not a clear cause for the seizure, then it's possible your child could have another seizure.

Q. *"But what caused the seizure?"*
A. After many first seizures, the doctor will respond, "I don't know." They may say, "It was idiopathic" (that's medicine's big word for "I don't know the cause"). In some cases, even after a first seizure, the doctor may be able to suspect a particular syndrome, especially if an EEG shows a specific pattern.

Physicians are uncomfortable saying, "I don't know." They are trained to search for reasons, for causes, so that they can treat or eliminate the cause. That is why, after a first seizure, many physicians will do various tests—an EEG, CT scans, MRI scans, blood and urine tests—to look for evidence of a specific syndrome or structural, chemical, or metabolic imbalances. These tests should probably be done on an individualized basis, depending on when the seizure happened, the type of seizure, and whether the child has returned to a completely normal baseline. Only when most possibilities have been exhausted, maybe even when "an expert" neurologist also cannot find a cause, is the doctor willing to accept "I don't know."

Parents are also frustrated with "I don't know." Medicine has oversold its ability to find causes. Until all the tests are done, and all the experts seen, many parents remain anxious, fearing the worst, and are unwilling to accept the concept that the cause is unknown.

In more than half of children with seizures in childhood, no cause can be found. Under these circumstances, it is understandable for a parent to be very anxious. We emphasize to parents that the best thing is to *not* to find a cause. It is *best* if the seizures are idiopathic. *Idiopathic* means there is no known cause, although we are beginning to think that these may be genetically determined, and terminology is beginning to change. The *known* causes of seizures are tumor, infections, structural problems, vascular problems, metabolic causes, genetic abnormalities, and trauma. In these cases, seizures are less likely to be outgrown.

- Seizures of unknown cause are the least likely to recur.

- Seizures of unknown cause are the most likely to be controlled with medication.

- Seizures of unknown cause are the most likely to be outgrown, even if they do recur.

- Sixty to 70 percent of seizures in childhood are idiopathic.

- Only half of first idiopathic seizures ever recur.

Q. *"Will my child be intellectually disabled?"*
A. No! A single tonic-clonic seizure does not cause intellectual disability or brain damage. We don't have evidence that recurrent seizures themselves cause intellectual disability or brain damage. It is true that tonic-clonic and other seizures occur more often among children who already have learning problems, brain dysfunction, brain damage, or intellectual disability, but there is no evidence that seizures make these conditions worse. *Most* children with such problems do not have seizures, and *most* children who have seizures do not have these problems.

Of course, you are afraid that seizures will recur, but try not to let this anxiety control your life or your child's life. It's okay for your child to do the things they did before without constant supervision.

If seizures do recur, most likely they will recur within two to three months after the first seizure. It might be reasonable to be a bit more cautious during this brief period. Maybe your child shouldn't be climbing trees or be in other potentially dangerous situations during this time. But there's no reason they can't swim like any other child with supervision, play most sports, go on field trips, and lead an otherwise normal life. If they were driving, they should stop for a few months and let the local motor vehicle association know.

What Do You Tell Your Child after a Single Seizure?

Be truthful and be simple. What you should tell your child depends on your child's age, sophistication, and level of understanding. It is always best to be honest. Otherwise, sooner or later, you may get trapped in a web of lies and cover-ups that will only make things worse. If your child does not ask questions, they may be too frightened and unable to articulate this fear. So, don't take their silence as meaning they have no concerns. Remember that your child probably has no memory of the event that was so frightening to you. Their first memory is likely to be of awakening in the ambulance or in the hospital emergency room. They are likely to be frightened because they don't know what happened—and are as fearful now of the unknown as you were.

To a young child, your explanation may be as simple as "You had something called a seizure. Something happened in your head, and you couldn't talk to me for a few minutes, and Mommy and Daddy got very excited and called the doctor, but they say that you're fine. And see, you're perfectly okay and talking to me now."

For an older child, you might talk about what a seizure is, about how the brain works based on electricity, and tell them that a seizure is like a sudden interruption in that circuitry that leads to something like static when your radio sounds fuzzy in a tunnel or an interruption on a TV program. The preteenager or teenager needs a more in-depth explanation. Your doctor or a nurse could do this, but you should discuss it with your child as well. They have heard about seizures and may have many misunderstandings. Give your child a chance to ask questions. Contact your local epilepsy organization or the national Epilepsy Foundation to get some publications geared to their age.

Explain that while there is no guarantee that a similar episode will not occur, many people never have another seizure. They are still your wonderful boy or girl, and everything is fine now. Be truthful and reassuring. Let them know that you were scared, too, but that when you understood what had happened, you were much less afraid.

What Do You Tell Other Children after a Single Seizure?

Using the same criteria we've discussed above about age appropriateness, reassure your other children. Brothers and sisters need to understand what happened, why you were upset, why you may be treating their brother or sister differently, and whether it will ever happen to them. Friends and playmates or schoolmates may or may not need to know, depending on whether they witnessed the seizure. If they did, you may obviously need to explain. You probably should check with their parents about how to approach them. You need to reassure them that their friend is all right and that they can't catch a seizure as if it were a cold. If friends didn't see the seizure happen, you should consider the pros and cons of telling them about something that may never happen again. Remember that your child may tell them something on their own.

What Do You Tell Relatives and Friends after a Single Seizure?

What you tell relatives and friends depends on many factors. There is no right answer. After a single seizure in a child who is otherwise well, you might decide to tell them nothing. Or you might decide to give them the same frank, simple explanation that you give to older children. The most frightening thing about seizures is the uncertainty. At this stage no one knows if or when they will recur. This frightening anticipation of the unknown is often far worse than the reality of a second seizure itself.

There is something to be gained and something to be lost by discussing the seizure with family and friends. Saying nothing may prevent some overprotection and the constant observation and anxiety. But informing them about the seizure may enable them to cope better should another seizure occur. Reassurance that seizures are common, often benign, not life threatening, and do not necessarily indicate a brain tumor or any other bad disease of the brain may be an important ingredient in helping your child lead a normal life.

What you tell others depends on who the others are, their relationships to you and your child, and the frequency of their contact—and their personalities. You will have to use your own judgment, but, in general, we prefer openness.

What Do You Tell the School after a Single Seizure?

In the best of all possible worlds, clearly you would tell the school about the seizure. Unfortunately, this is not the best of worlds. Prejudice, misconceptions, overconcern, and fear of seizures still exist. Therefore, there is no simple correct answer to the question. In general, there is no need to tell the school about a single seizure. There is nothing school officials can do, or should do, about your child. They need not watch them more carefully unless they are participating in gymnastics that would place them at heights or are swimming. Schools should not restrict them from playing on sports teams or at recess. Your child should be allowed to go on field trips and to do everything the other children do.

Since there is nothing special school personnel need to do after a single seizure, it may not be necessary to let them know about it. What or whether you tell the school about the seizure may depend on your assessment of the teacher, the principal, and the school nurse and how you think they will react to the information. If your son or daughter does have another seizure, and if it occurs in school, you will wish that you had told them if you did not. After a second or third tonic-clonic seizure, or with epilepsy, it's a different matter, which we discuss later in this chapter.

This same philosophy applies to day care and to babysitters. Individuals acting as surrogate parents should have the same information and philosophy about overprotection you have.

Schoolteachers and school administrators are apprehensive about what they don't know or understand. In today's lawsuit-prone society, they are even more nervous. This is why we don't necessarily recommend telling them about a single seizure. The same is true for day care workers, babysitters, sports coaches, and others who come in transient contact with your child. Although there could be another seizure, and you might wish that you had told them in advance, remember there is a great chance that another seizure will never occur.

Q. *"My stepfather [or mother, aunt, etc.] thinks that I should get another opinion. What do you think?"*
A. Your physician should never be hesitant about referring you to another physician for a second opinion if you think it would be helpful with

your ability to cope. If they are hesitant, then we would recommend that you get another physician. Nonetheless, after a single seizure is probably not a time to get a second opinion. There is general consensus among physicians that no treatment is needed at this point in children. If your child doesn't need medication or further testing, and you don't need to place any significant restrictions on your child, then a second opinion isn't going to tell you anything you don't already know. But sometimes hearing it again can be reassuring. If your child has another seizure, or if there are other things about your child that are of concern, then talk further with your child's physician. Perhaps they can be of help, or perhaps they can recommend a specialist in your area of concern.

Recurrent Seizures: Epilepsy

If the first seizure wasn't a tonic-clonic episode or didn't involve a loss of consciousness or fall to the ground, then by the time you recognize that recurring episodes (absence, focal seizures, etc.) are seizures, epilepsy is present. If tonic-clonic seizures do recur, your response will be different from your reaction after the first seizure. You have already been through the initial shock of seeing tonic-clonic shaking. You may have come to terms with your initial anxiety. Hopefully you know what to do this second time and are less frightened than at first. But you may be discouraged. Your hopes that a seizure would not recur have been dashed. What is worse, your child's physician has now used the word *epilepsy*. Although *epilepsy* simply means recurrent seizures, the term still carries a lot of baggage—myths, stigma, and prejudices—as we discuss earlier in this book. And it means that you need to be sure that other issues, such as learning and psychological functioning, are addressed.

When many people think of epilepsy, they think of the child who is severely handicapped by continuing seizures. Yet those children are a small subgroup of children with epilepsy. The largest group are those with *benign epilepsy of childhood*, who have seizures that can be controlled with medicines and that are often outgrown. In most children with epilepsy (six or seven out of ten), seizures can be controlled— yes, completely controlled. When a child's epilepsy is under control, it shouldn't significantly alter their life or yours. The myths are wrong!

For about 30 percent of children with epilepsy, however, seizures may be difficult to control. Control will require using different medications or treatments, coping with their side effects, and perhaps even surgery. If your child has difficult-to-control epilepsy, your life and your child's life are obviously going to change in significant ways.

Which group will your child fit into? After only a second or even after a third tonic-clonic seizure, it may be difficult to tell. We are beginning to be able to predict this, as we indicate in Chapter 9. Predictions are based on the cause, the nature of the seizures, and often the EEG.

Absence Seizures

If your child has staring spells, or absence seizures—instances when they briefly stop and stare, perhaps with some smacking of the lips, picking at clothes, or confusion—the chances are that they have not had just a single episode. These brief spells are usually diagnosed only after many have occurred. Since it is likely that you are recognizing the problem after the fifth, the tenth, or the hundredth spell, it is obvious that the spells are likely to continue, to recur, unless treated with medication.

While less frightening than the tonic-clonic seizure, staring spells cause a particular type of anxiety. Parents are worried that they won't even know when their child is having a seizure. "Is Jane just daydreaming, as all children do, or is she having an absence seizure?" "Should I have yelled at George for not taking out the garbage? Did he not hear me? Did he disobey, or was he having an absence seizure?" Since these seizures are brief and subtle and therefore difficult to recognize, it is probably even more important to tell neighbors, friends, grandparents, and the school about them. This awareness will permit other people to notice when they occur, to be more tolerant of "daydreaming," and to be a bit more careful when the child is crossing the street or in a situation where loss of awareness could cause harm. Also, because this type of seizure is likely to occur far more frequently than tonic-clonic seizures (sometimes many times each day or several times per week), staring spells are *more* likely than the single tonic-clonic seizure to interfere with the child's functioning.

Again, it is important to be truthful, but since the child will likely be unaware of these spells unless someone tells them, the explanation needs to be handled with sensitivity. "You have short episodes when you don't know what is going on. They're like interference on the TV, a brief second or two when you lose the picture and sound for a moment. And then the cable service is quickly restored." It is important to use terms appropriate for the age and understanding of the child and to make sure that the words you use are not frightening. Better for you to tell them than for them to be asked awkward questions or be told disturbing stories by other children.

You need to give your child the opportunity to let you know they're missing things in school—for example, instructions or the end of a story. We know of one child who assumed that life was just a series of blank spaces. His class was making a movie about a train going by, and he wanted to cut out pieces of the film. When asked why, he told his teacher that's how he saw it—with short blank spots between the pictures. It was then that his teacher became aware that there were frequent, very brief, gaps in his attention. The diagnosis of absence seizures was eventually made.

These simple absence seizures can usually be brought completely under control with medication, although it may take several weeks to gain control. Until then, the child's activities should be more carefully supervised, with caution and concern but without overprotectiveness or panic.

Teachers are an important, perhaps even crucial, part of the evaluation and treatment of a child who has absence seizures. School classes are one of the few times when a child is consistently under observation and when brief lapses in attention can be readily recognized. It is not uncommon for the teacher to be the first to recognize these lapses of attention. Some parents feel guilty that they did not notice these lapses themselves, but in the structured atmosphere of the classroom, they are often easier to see and recognize than in the more informal atmosphere of a family. And once they are recognized, the teacher can be your child's best ally, by noting spells and possible side effects of medication.

On the other hand, because of the myths about epilepsy, an uninformed or biased teacher may begin to treat your child as if they had a learning problem or were stupid. Normal daydreaming may be misperceived as staring spells. A child who is daydreaming may or may not respond if called on but will certainly respond if the teacher goes over and touches them. When a child does not respond when touched, they are more likely to be experiencing absence seizures.

Focal Unaware Seizures

In focal unaware seizures (previously called complex partial seizures), as with absence seizures, the child stops, stares, and is unaware of their environment. But in this case, there is often a period of confusion after the child stops staring. Also, during the episode, they may get up and wander around the room, pick at their clothes, and fail to respond appropriately. These peculiar episodes are likely to be misunderstood by the other children in a classroom and by their teachers. As with absence spells, it is important that the teacher understand what is happening. The teacher needs to realize that if your child is wandering around, perhaps someone should close the door so they can't leave the room or move things out of the way so that they can't harm themselves. That is usually better than trying to restrain them, since the child may lash out and even become highly agitated. Providing gentle guidance and supervision at such times is far better than trying to force them to sit down. The teacher needs to be able to be comforting and reassuring both to the student having the seizure, who is not aware of what is happening, and to the other children, who may be confused by the behavior. It is important that the teacher alert you to changes in your child's performance. You can then alert your child's doctor.

As with other recurrent seizures, your child needs to understand what is happening during these episodes when they are not aware. They may remember the beginning of the seizure; they may feel an aura (for example, fear or a rising feeling in the stomach), and they may be vaguely aware of people responding to their behavior during and after the seizure. Or they may be aware only that something happened and that now things are different from what they were a few seconds or minutes ago. Since these spells usually follow a pattern, let them know what has been going on, so that they will be less upset and confused. If they do have an aura, point out that it can be a useful warning. Encourage them to pay attention to it, so that they can avoid harmful situations when a seizure may be coming on.

Benign Epilepsy of Childhood

Once upon a time, epilepsy was considered a chronic disease. People who had two or more seizures were declared to have epilepsy, and it was believed that they were destined to have seizures forever. The real situation now is quite different:

- Seventy percent of children whose seizures are controlled for two years can go off medication and remain seizure-free. These children have either outgrown their epilepsy or have been "cured."

- Only one in five children who have one tonic-clonic seizure and a normal EEG will have a second seizure, whether or not they are treated.

- Children who are otherwise developmentally normal, who have no evidence of prior damage or dysfunction of the brain, are likely to outgrow their epilepsy.

Benign epilepsy of childhood is a new concept, one not universally accepted, but one we are convinced by observation really exists. Our conviction is reinforced by the fact that the threshold for seizures increases as the young child's brain matures, and they are more resistant to seizures, and also by the fact that genetic tendencies toward seizures are influenced by age—most children outgrow their epilepsy.

How do you know if your child has benign epilepsy of childhood? After a second seizure, neither you nor your child's doctor can be sure, but if your child is neurologically and developmentally normal, and if the EEG does not show abnormalities, then there is good reason to hope. Only time will tell.

Stages of Acceptance

Parents go through many stages of acceptance when their child is diagnosed with epilepsy, and it is important to realize this early in the process. They do not always occur in a particular order, and they are often revisited when something changes.

Fear is parents' *normal* response to hearing that their child has epilepsy. You are fearful because of your concerns about what epilepsy might do. You fear that the seizures may present difficulties: you will now have to take time to go to the doctor; it will interfere with your job, your activities, your interests. You fear that your child's life—and your life—have changed forever. This is really fear of the unknown. Information helps make the unknown known. Reality is always less frightening than what you imagine. A child can often sense fear, and good explanations of what has happened are critical to the child's well-being.

Grief is another emotion that parents must go through when faced with epilepsy. You are sad and you grieve for the child who you think no longer exists as before. You grieve for yourself because you're embarrassed and fearful. All these feelings are common and normal. Indeed, we worry about the parent who shows no signs of grieving. You have to go through grief before you can achieve acceptance.

How do you cope with this grief? It's all right to cry, to feel sorry for yourself and your child. You need to realize that you may not be able to cope alone. Grieving is much easier when it is shared with someone else. Another person can help you put your grief in perspective. You need to reach out and find support. You may find this within your own home, by talking about your fears and concerns with a member of the family. You may find it from another parent or group of parents. The Epilepsy Foundation or your local affiliate may be able to put you in touch with resources that will help you deal with these feelings. Fortunately, many online resources are now being made available to families through these organizations. This is particularly true if your child has a specific type or cause of epilepsy. There is a wonderful, comprehensive report with many resources provided by the Institute of Medicine ("Quality of Life and Community Resources," in *Epilepsy Across the Spectrum*, https://www.ncbi.nlm.nih.gov/books/NBK100593/). In addition, many parent support groups exist and can be helpful. You should ask your child's doctor if there is a specific organization that may be of help to you.

Anger is often the next stage. You're angry because the ambulance took so long to come, angry that the emergency room was so crowded and inefficient, angry that the nurse was not more considerate, and angry that the doctor didn't take more time examining your child and explaining things to you. You are angry at the system and the world, at your partner because they are not more concerned or involved or are too concerned and involved, angry at yourself for being angry. You may even be angry at your child, even though you know the seizure was not their fault and that your anger is irrational.

Again, all these reactions are perfectly normal. Different people handle them differently and at varying speeds. Your partner may be at a different stage than you are. They may be more fearful and not yet have progressed to the stage of grieving or anger. Occasionally a person moves through these stages rapidly, but more often it takes weeks and sometimes months; eventually you will get through them. You can deal with anger in many of the same ways you managed to deal with grief. Talking to others may help you to put your anger in perspective. Communication between parents can be difficult; your partner may not understand your feelings. You may resent a seeming insensitivity. Openness and communication are the only way to deal with these feelings of anger. You may need someone to help you find a way to talk with your partner about your feelings.

Anger is often long lasting, but it can be made productive. If you're angry at the school because of their attitude toward your child, perhaps the best way to handle it is to educate the school system, so that they may treat the next child better. If you're angry at your child's doctor, it may be important to discuss with them why you are angry. Discuss what they said, or what they didn't say, that made you upset. Sometimes your doctor may have said things that were inappropriate, but often parents misunderstand what physicians say or mean to say. Communication is always difficult, particularly in times of stress. Talking should improve matters.

Anger, of itself, is not productive. A person who continues to be angry ultimately alienates those who could be supportive.

Acceptance also takes time. It, too, has many different stages. Sometimes using the power of positive thinking can be helpful, and we discuss it more extensively in Chapter 24. Some parents would like to deny that a seizure ever occurred. These parents might say, "It won't happen again, and I won't let the seizure affect my life or my child's life." But it did occur, and it may recur, and it did affect your life. Whatever approach you take—and different individuals take different approaches—all these phases should eventually lead to acceptance.

Acceptance means that you can consider your child a wonderful child who happens to have seizures. It means realizing that your child is not "an epileptic." Lack of acceptance, by comparison, can lead to overprotection, overpermissiveness, lack of discipline, and an inability to set appropriate limits for your child.

Communicating with Others

Parents are typically the people who have to communicate with several people about a child's epilepsy. This involves having a good grasp of the nature of your child's seizures and how they are affecting their life.

Brothers and Sisters

Sibling love, as well as sibling rivalry, is normal. The reaction of a child's brother or sister to a sibling with epilepsy will depend on age and developmental stage but most of all on your reaction to epilepsy and to each of your children.

All children fantasize, and it is not uncommon for children to believe that they caused their sibling's seizures by playing with them roughly or pushing them and causing a fall. Children often wish for something bad to happen to their brother or sister. If something does happen, then guilt is a common response. These feelings may be compounded by jealousy because you are giving so much attention to the child who has seizures. Brothers and sisters may show these feelings by acting out, by withdrawing, or by displaying signs of depression, any of which may affect the sibling's school performance and sleep patterns.

Children often believe that epilepsy, like the flu or COVID, is contagious and that they might catch it, too. This fear should be discussed openly within the family. In families where there is a strong genetic predisposition for epilepsy, you may want to enlist the help of a genetic counselor experienced in working with children since it is possible that other siblings or relatives may at some point have a seizure as well.

Your other children may also be drawn into a pattern of overprotection or overindulgence. Either you or they may say, "Don't play so roughly; you might bring on a seizure." "Don't let him get so excited." "Give him the toy, or he'll get upset and have a seizure." Such statements give enormous leverage to children with epilepsy to manipulate the people around them.

Most of these problems can be avoided by your sensitivity to the effects of your child's epilepsy on their brothers and sisters. The siblings of children with epilepsy may feel invisible at times, particularly if the affected sibling has multiple complex health care needs. It is important that you initiate discussions with your other children and find some time to spend individually with them. No matter how time consuming and preoccupying your child's seizure problems may be, expressing your continued love for all your children by talking and doing something special with them and for them is crucial.

While there is always an impact on siblings whose brother or sister has a disability, studies have shown that, if handled appropriately, the impact is positive. Brothers and sisters can become stronger, more sympathetic, more empathetic, and more caring.

We have found one other way to be helpful to siblings of a child with epilepsy.

Sibling Workshops

Sibshops, as they are sometimes called, meet periodically under the leadership of the local Epilepsy Foundation affiliate and often meet online. The Sibshops are led by a person who is well versed in epilepsy and its effects and adept at working with children and adolescents. Sibshops allow the siblings of a child with epilepsy to talk about the problems of having a brother or sister who seems to get more than their share of attention, who requires special attention, who doesn't do an equal share of the chores, who may receive less discipline and more praise. Many of these complaints are common to all siblings, even when there are no medical problems in the brother or sister, but these feelings are stronger in siblings of children who do indeed require different care. These types of sibling workshops often exist for other developmental disabilities as well, like autism, intellectual disability, and cerebral palsy.

Allowing siblings to talk about their problems and their perceptions, to hear that others are facing difficulties also, and to find out how others have coped with them can only be of benefit. Brainstorming about solutions is also helpful. Every child thinks that they are the only one to have suffered such a fate. Such discussions can be invaluable, particularly when led by a good counselor.

At times, older siblings are given undue responsibility for the child with epilepsy or other disabilities. This is often true when the affected sibling has multiple handicaps. It is important to recognize when this extra responsibility is becoming burdensome for the sibling, and to be sensitive to the responsibilities placed on a youth or adolescent. Keep the lines of communication open and be ready to help siblings avoid or solve problems.

What Do You Tell Relatives and Your Friends?

When your child has had a second or third seizure, family and friends need to be informed. Your child has probably been started on medication and could experience side effects or even temporary changes in personality from the medication. The likelihood that your child will have another seizure is now high enough that those close to them should be aware of the situation. They should know what these frightening episodes look like and what they should do if another occurs. They should have the various myths about epilepsy dispelled. Most of the time your child will be normal. Make sure their epilepsy is not blown out of proportion. Don't let your friends and relatives dwell on it. If they understand, perhaps they can help avoid the overprotection and inappropriate restrictions that deprive your child of normal experiences.

The Child's Friends

It is up to you and your child to tell their friends about their epilepsy. The information conveyed, and the persons to whom it is conveyed, should depend on the type and frequency of the seizures. For the child with absence or focal unaware seizures that occur with some frequency, it is far better for the friend to understand the seizures than to assume that they are "weird," "on drugs," or "going crazy." One of our teenagers with unrecognized absence seizures had been nicknamed Spacey by her friends. It is more useful for a friend to understand what to do should a seizure occur and not to panic.

Unless the seizures are frequent, it is unnecessary to inform everyone with whom your child comes in contact. Their good friends and those families with whom they spend time, however, should be aware of their seizures and how they are controlled. In general, the fears and apprehensions that result from ignorance are far worse than any reality.

"Should I tell my date?" is a question teenagers often ask us. Again, this depends on the frequency and type of the seizures. Certainly, if a relationship begins to become serious, your teenager should be self-confident enough to talk openly about their condition.

What Do You Tell the School and Classmates?

Teachers are an important part of your child's environment and can be enormously helpful to a child with epilepsy. If they are informed and properly educated, teachers will know what to do and what to say to classmates should a seizure occur in school. They need to be prepared should a tonic-clonic seizure occur. They need to know what your child's seizures look like so they can inform you if there is recurrence. They can be helpful in alerting the parent and physician to changes in performance or personality that might be related to drug toxicity.

One of the prevailing myths is that children with epilepsy are stupid or have learning problems. According to many studies, children with epilepsy do tend to have more difficulties in school, but this may be a consequence of fear or anxiety, their own and others. This does not mean that all children with epilepsy have learning problems. Most children with epilepsy do not. Some teachers may see learning problems that aren't there. They may be responding to the myths. But often, the teacher is sensitive to your child's needs. If they point out problems, your child's physician can evaluate whether they are related to medication. If the problems aren't due to medication, it may be helpful to have neuropsychological testing done. The school needs to devise an individual educational program to meet your child's needs if one is required.

Learning problems may not be the result of epilepsy at all. Many children who never had epilepsy don't learn easily. Or, as noted, problems may be a side effect of medication. A change in your child's personality or in their abilities when medication is started may signal such a cause. Early identification of this possibility may allow the physician either to reduce the dose of the drug or to change the medication (see Chapter 10).

To be sure that teachers, school nurses, and principals have accurate information about epilepsy, you may provide some of the excellent pamphlets or links to internet sites available either directly from the Epilepsy Foundation or from a local affiliate. Many pamphlets are written so that a young child can understand them and are available either free or for only a nominal charge. Pamphlets that explain epilepsy in simple terms can be given to a young child's siblings and friends and, when appropriate, can be used in the child's classroom. Your local epilepsy association can probably provide speakers or perhaps the wonderful puppet show *Kids on the Block* and will try to help educate the school. A brief classroom session may help your child's classmates be more understanding, helpful, and friendly should they see your child have a seizure. There is a lot of help out there, but you have to ask for it.

Working with Others

Some families can take a different approach and want to help others outside their family, or even help advance public health. There are many ways you can do this. First, ask your epilepsy team if there are support groups through the hospital or ways to teach new families about epilepsy or a treatment. Most hospitals have development officers who are willing to discuss ways in which families can help support research and advocacy. New families are anxious to meet families that have been through this before; a quick email or phone call with support to say "you're not alone" can go a long way. Second, there may be regional support groups, such as the local chapter of the Epilepsy Foundation or charities. Finally, on a national level, there are groups such as Cure Epilepsy, the Epilepsy Foundation, and organizations focusing on a condition or treatment (e.g., Charlie Foundation [ketogenic diet], Glut1 Deficiency Foundation, Hemispherectomy Foundation) that are always looking for new parents to help with conferences and fundraising. In many of these examples, the child can help as well as the parents.

CHAPTER 24

Psychological Strategies

Coping, Resilience, and Counseling

It is generally understood that epilepsy is a medical disorder of the brain. But as anyone whose life has been touched by epilepsy can tell you, it is so much more than intermittent electrical misfiring that causes seizures. Epilepsy, like many chronic conditions, has a profound impact on all aspects of life. Seizures are usually unpredictable. They can occur at any time and sometimes with little warning. Unlike other chronic health conditions, which may affect life in a fairly consistent way, recurrent seizures often wax and wane, with periods of relative quiet being punctuated with sometimes sudden and often inconvenient seizures. People with epilepsy and their loved ones often find it difficult to ever fully let their guard down and may be left wondering "when the other shoe is going to drop." For this reason, the psychosocial impact of epilepsy can be equal to or greater than the physical toll of the condition on patients and families. Therefore, the treatment of epilepsy would not be complete without addressing its psychosocial aspects.

In the previous edition of this book, we stated that psychological dysfunction was not *intrinsic* to epilepsy. And while it is true that seizures themselves do not necessarily cause psychological problems like depression, we now know that the relationship between mood and epilepsy is complex. While we still have much to learn, it's likely that epilepsy and mood disorders share similar biological and chemical pathways in the brain, suggesting that the underlying cause may be linked. In addition, the psychosocial impact of epilepsy is affected by the reactions, or perceived reactions, of others to persons with epilepsy, as well as the reaction of the person with epilepsy to their own diagnosis. These reactions play a crucial role in coping and, more important, resilience. Let's break this down a little more.

Parent Coping and Resilience

As a parent, having your child receive a diagnosis of epilepsy is like being punched in the gut. Regardless of whether it was unexpected or simply confirmed what you already knew, the finality of hearing the diagnosis spoken aloud is immensely difficult. There are many reasons for this. First, the stigma that surrounds an epilepsy diagnosis remains undeniable. Many parents' thoughts jump to worst-case scenarios, imagining their child permanently and devastatingly disabled, never able to have a "normal" life. (This is known as *catastrophizing*.) While this response is completely understandable and typical, it is often not true; multiple, ongoing honest discussions with your child's neurologist can generally clear up the myths and misunderstandings that surround an epilepsy diagnosis and allow parents to move forward with a more accurate picture of what challenges their child will realistically face. But sometimes it is impossible for your doctor to honestly predict the future and how well your child's seizures will respond to treatment.

As time goes on, the uncertainty that inevitably accompanies an epilepsy diagnosis can take a toll. Children and their families often find themselves constantly on edge, awaiting the next seizure. *When will it happen? Where will it be? Will I be there to help my child when they need me? Will my child be okay?* It's hard to get too comfortable when you are worried that everything can suddenly and unexpectedly change because of a seizure.

You may wonder why parent coping is being addressed before child coping. Doesn't epilepsy primarily affect the child? Yes and no. Epilepsy doesn't just affect a person; if affects entire families, sometimes entire communities. As a parent, your child's feelings about and ability to cope with the diagnosis are inextricably intertwined with yours, and it is important for you to be aware of your own thoughts and feelings regarding the epilepsy diagnosis, both initially and as time goes on. This is not to say that you must immediately and unconditionally accept the diagnosis and all that it entails, but you must be willing to continually pause and reflect on what is going on in your own mind.

Q. *"What am I thinking? What am I feeling? What judgments am I making about myself or my child? What distorted or irrational thoughts am I having?"*
A. It is important to keep in mind that your reactions to your child's diagnosis, on some level, will guide your child's reactions. Your beliefs, for better or worse, integrate into your children's beliefs about themselves. It's important to be aware of the messages we send, even unknowingly. Being aware of your own feelings and being willing to accept them as is, without judgment, will ultimately help you accept your child as well. Self-acceptance allows space for empathy when interacting with your child. It will promote open communication by allowing you to validate their feelings and helping them to feel understood. The ultimate goal is that children feel competent to manage their emotions and circumstances independently and to learn to successfully adapt to the stress of life events. This, of course, is the definition of resilience.

The Power of Reshaping Thinking

When your child has had one seizure, and even when a child has been diagnosed as having epilepsy, it is important for you and your child that you both develop a positive approach, to reshape the way in which you are thinking about the issues. One way to achieve a positive approach to dealing with this uncertainty is to focus on the low probability of another seizure. A second way is to recognize that another seizure may occur, accept that possibility, and know that there is a plan in place to deal with it. Find what approach works for you and your child, what approach leads to less anxiety and acceptance.

You might say to yourself: "She's going to be one of the lucky ones with benign epilepsy who will, or has, outgrown it." Or you might say, "Chances are that she will never have another seizure." Never is a long time, though, and it might be more useful to say, "She's not going to have another seizure today." If you said that to yourself, the chances are overwhelming that you would be correct. If you said, "I don't think she will have another seizure this week or this month," you still have an enormous chance of being right. Many people with epilepsy have only two, or three, or four seizures in their lifetimes.

What happens if your confidence is wrong, and your child has another seizure? You and your child's physician will explore why that seizure occurred. Did your child forget their medicine? Not get enough sleep? Do they have an infection? Does the medication need adjusting? You may find a good reason. If you don't, you will have to begin your positive, reshaped thinking all over again.

Yet, you'll be right about her not having a seizure far more often than you'll be wrong. And since the consequences of being wrong are not within your control, this framework may help you and your child achieve a more positive approach to living.

Another approach involves the realization that the medical risks of a recurrent seizure are minimal and that, as in the past, your child will quickly recover from the seizure and resume her normal activities. You may even be able to accept the social consequences and not be overly concerned that you or your child will experience embarrassment. It may be easier for your child to do this if they have a good understanding of seizures and if you have been able to educate their school and their friends that, although having a seizure is unpleasant and interrupts activities for a short while, these activities usually can be resumed without any real harm. This approach is realistic when an "if this, then that" strategy is in place. It involves recognizing that a seizure might happen, but that it's important to live as normally as possible in all the time in between.

Child Coping and Resilience

As a parent, helping your child cope effectively with an epilepsy diagnosis is crucial; you are a key part of your child's emotional guidance system. While your child's physician will take the lead in managing the seizures, building resilience will be the work of the child's caregivers. This is tremendously important work. An epilepsy diagnosis has the potential to wreak havoc on a child's or teenager's sense of autonomy, independence, and identity. They may question their abilities or worth. As a parent, you can serve as an anchor.

The Child's Self-Perception

Self-image and self-esteem are important ingredients of success in later life. How does your child's self-image change after a seizure? The answer to this may depend on their self-image before the seizure. The change, if any, will depend on the type of seizure and its immediate effects on them, on their developmental age, and on what, if anything, follows the seizure. Most important, self-image and self-esteem will depend on how your child and the seizure are treated by you, by your friends and family, and by your child's doctor.

The response of family and friends is perhaps the principal determinant of the eventual outcome for the young child, and for children of all ages, your response is the principal factor under your control.

Accurate and honest information that is presented in an age-appropriate way appears to be an important ingredient of any child's self-perception. This has been best documented in adolescents. In many studies, the adolescents who were the least informed were the ones with the poorest psychosocial adjustment. The quality of their adjustment did not correlate with their seizure control or with their neurological normalcy. The adolescents who were most physically normal—who had no neurological abnormality and whose seizures were under control—often were most negative about their social adjustment.

A key factor in nurturing your child's resilience is helping them regain a sense of control of their lives, particularly after an event, like a diagnosis of epilepsy, that has likely left them feeling powerless. Encouraging your child to participate in discussions about their epilepsy and its treatment allows them to pivot from a position of powerlessness, a person who is at the mercy of both a disease and the doctors who treat it, to an active decision maker, someone who is taking control of their own destiny. Which narrative is more empowering?

Most of these psychosocial problems can be prevented if your child is included in discussions of their epilepsy and its treatment. Having age-appropriate discussions with your child about epilepsy, their particular type of seizures, and the reason for taking medication is an important first step in their understanding and accepting the condition. In one study, it was revealed that many children still believed they could swallow their tongues during a seizure. They feared that they might die. Unfounded apprehensions seem to be more damaging than the reality. Shielding your child from the facts to prevent them from being scared is more likely to lead to worse, but unspoken, fears than are honesty and openness.

Your attitude toward your child and their seizures will affect their own attitude. If you are frightened, they may be too, even if they don't understand why. If you are overprotective, they may respond by becoming either dependent or rebellious. Your understanding that they are normal most of the time and your honest calmness will allow them to get on with the process of developing independence and competence.

It should be the job of your child's physician and the rest of the therapeutic team to be sure that issues of honesty, overprotection, and dependency are discussed with you and your partner and that you come to terms with them. The epilepsy team should also discuss the seizures, medication, and reasonable restrictions with your child and make sure that you have also discussed them with your child in age-appropriate terms.

Remember that ultimately, epilepsy is your child's problem. If the seizures continue or if they must continue to take medication, then they will have to assume responsibility for their condition and its treatment. If your child is given a sense of control from the beginning, they will feel more responsible for their future life. We try to have these discussions with children when they are as young as 5 or 6 years. Responsibility clearly increases with age, but participation can rarely begin too early.

Helping Your Child Cope with Epilepsy

Your child will go through the same emotional stages you do. The manifestations of these stages will vary with the child's age and maturity and with the kind of seizures involved. They will also vary based on your ability to deal with your own emotions.

Fear or anxiety is real for many of these children. Children may fear dying even if they have no concept of death. This fear of dying should be dealt with forthrightly. All people fear losing control, and people who have seizures are made anxious by the fact that a seizure could happen at any time. In fact, this anticipation (and not knowing when their life will be interrupted again) may be the most disabling psychological stress. Educating your child about what actually happens during their seizures, what they look like to others, and reassuring them that they will always return to their previous normal state may help them adjust to this fear. For the older child, the fear of embarrassment may be even worse than the fear of death. "What will my friends think of me? Suppose I wet myself? Suppose this happens at a dance or in school?" Acceptance by one's peers is critical in adolescence. The worst thing that can happen to most teens is that somebody will notice that they are different.

Helping your child understand epilepsy and accept it to the point where they can explain it to their friends and classmates is the most important element in overcoming these fears.

Judy told us that seizures had ruined her life. She felt she no longer had friends. She had given up field hockey because she was afraid that a seizure might happen on the field. She now hated school. Even though her seizures had come under control, she was an unhappy young lady. We finally got her to begin to accept her epilepsy by encouraging her to tell the field hockey coach that she had seizures and that they were controlled. Getting her to go back out for the team was the first step in rebuilding her life. Since she could play with the team, she began to realize that she wasn't different from her teammates. As she felt better about herself, her schoolwork improved, and her attitude shifted. When she was able to tell classmates about the seizures and what it was like to feel different, Judy began to realize that the rest of the kids never really felt she was different. She realized that her isolation was self-imposed, constructed because she was worried that they might feel that she was different. Once she became aware that the problem was within her and not them, she could work to regain her self-esteem.

Grieving also occurs in children. Initially the older child or adolescent will think that life has ended, that they can no longer do the same things others are doing. If you impose unwarranted restrictions, your child will not be able to continue their usual activities, and they will lose a previous lifestyle; then there may truly be reason for grieving. This is one of the reasons it is so important that your child be allowed to participate in their chosen activities to the fullest extent possible. Even when restrictions are needed because of the frequency or severity of the seizures, it is important that you find activities in which your child can participate and achieve safely. Achievement and participation are important ingredients in helping people develop self-esteem.

Here are a couple of examples of how children can be helped through these stages of adjustment to having epilepsy:

• *Kamala was still grieving. This bright, articulate, theatrically talented teenager had had staring spells for almost nine months. Although she had been to many doctors, she was trying to deny that there was anything wrong, and she refused to take medicine. We were the ones who finally told her that she had epilepsy. Even though she had begun to take her medicine reliably and had had no seizures in two months, she felt sad. Seizures no longer interfered with any of her many activities, and there were no side effects from medication; but she still felt different, and she was still angry. We helped her move toward acceptance by offering her an opportunity to meet with other young people who had seizures, youngsters who had already been through some of these stages. We began to see a difference—a willingness to channel these feelings in a productive way. We saw a young lady who was beginning to believe that she was not handicapped by her seizures. Now, three years later, she has been abroad and is in college majoring in drama.*

• *Jackson felt sad. Although only 9, he had coped with his seizures by talking about them incessantly to all his classmates and friends. Unfortunately, this was not productive; it resulted in negative reactions. Most of his young peers didn't care, and so they ignored him or were angry at him for bothering them. We let Jackson know that lots of people have seizures. It had a profound impact on him when we told him that the Orioles' baseball stadium could be filled with people from Maryland who have epilepsy. Also, meeting another child with epilepsy who un-*

derstood his feelings made it possible for him to begin to put his seizures into perspective. He no longer feels alone.

Both of these children were grieving and had not accepted their epilepsy. Kamala had internalized the problem and withdrawn, while Jackson had externalized his difficulties and was making himself a nuisance. Neither response was productive.

Children, like the adults around them, ultimately need to accept their epilepsy if they are to be happy and productive citizens. They need to realize that epilepsy is only one part of their life and, for most children, not the dominant part. *People should be defined by the kind of person they are, not a condition they have.*

Perhaps most important to a child's acceptance of epilepsy is a feeling of self-esteem. For anyone to achieve their full potential, they must feel good about themselves and be able to achieve.

One aspect of self-esteem is a child's feeling of control over their epilepsy and their life. This is the reason children should participate in their treatment. Certainly, the older child must know why they are taking medicine. A parent who tells their child that they are taking medication because "It's good for you" or "It's a vitamin and will make you stronger" has not accepted the child's epilepsy and is not allowing the child to accept it either. Also, we encourage parents to let the child, from almost any age, be responsible for taking their own medication. The younger child will require supervision. The older child and adolescent can supervise themselves, or learn to, and in doing so, gain a feeling of control over their epilepsy. We realize that it is scary for parents not to make sure their child has taken their medicine, not to ask, not to hand it to them. But it is crucial that children learn responsibility. Often a pill case or perhaps an app on their phone can be helpful. They need to learn that it is their epilepsy, not yours, and that the consequences of not taking medicine are theirs, not yours—as much as you wish otherwise. This is the beginning of their ability to control the frightening uncertainties of their condition and of life.

An individual is known by what they can do, not by what they can't do. If you focus on your child's limitations and wish for things that are not realistic, your child is likely to become a failure in your eyes and in their own and may fail to achieve their potential. Recognizing your child's potential for achievement is a first step in helping them recognize their own capabilities. Rewarding achievement is far more productive than focusing on failure.

Overprotection and Overindulgence

Protection of their young is the natural reaction of parents. Even in the absence of disability, parents raising children must tread the fine line between protection and overprotection. The helicopter parent (hovering) generally is a disadvantage for a child. This line of protection changes with the age of the child and is challenged by the independent adult trying to emerge from the child during adolescence. Your natural reaction to protect your child is greatly magnified when they are injured or ill. You naturally want to protect them from the cruelties of the public and their peers. You want to shield them from further physical and emotional injury. Your overprotection is magnified by your anxieties, fears, and often by an unwarranted sense of guilt. These are normal reactions, but they may deprive your child of the rewards of having successfully coped with the challenges themselves.

It is important to remember to look inward and try to identify what concerns are reasonable and what thoughts are irrational or unrealistic. We do this by challenging irrational and unrealistic thinking through objectively evaluating the facts and the given situation.

Shantelle wanted to try out for cheerleading. It was very clear to her mother that her poorly controlled seizures and her general clumsiness would not allow her to make the squad. Rather than preventing her from competing, her mother helped Shantelle to realize that many people try out but are unsuccessful, and that while trying out was terrific, she needed to be able to cope with the possibility of not being selected. Her mother went to the tryouts and took a lot of pictures. Indeed, Shantelle did not make the squad, but she was thrilled to have been part of the process. She saw that many other wonderful girls didn't make it either. She was not terribly disappointed, and she had some wonderful memories for her scrapbook.

Growing up requires risks to achieve benefits. Your child with epilepsy, like any child, needs opportunities to achieve independence. Opportunities necessarily entail risks. Think carefully about how much the epilepsy has really increased your child's risk.

The other side of overprotection is overindulgence. It can be equally destructive. "But if I yell at him, he might have a seizure." "He throws a tantrum when he doesn't get his own way, and I don't want to upset him." "She's been through so much; I don't want to keep her from . . ." We hear these types of statements from many parents. When the seizures are subsequently brought under control with medication, these parents are left with a spoiled, undisciplined child or adolescent who is not handicapped by epilepsy but is socially handicapped.

Counseling

In the original editions of this book, our counselor Diana Pillas provided the insights to this subject that she had learned and practiced over decades working with patients and families. Sadly, her voice is lost to us, but the principles that she practiced and the advice that she offered in this book live on. Unfortunately, the realities of medicine today also make it difficult financially for practitioners and clinics to offer these visits in the clinical setting. Time and billing often don't allow for it. Families need to look for settings that find ways to provide counseling or at least guidance and help in finding resources where it can be provided. These might include the Epilepsy Foundation, local therapists who are knowledgeable about epilepsy, or perhaps online groups.

Guidance and counseling, commonly used as synonymous terms, have somewhat different connotations to us. Guidance is something one person, usually an expert, provides to another. It implies, to us at least, something actively given and passively received. It is typically preventive. Counseling, on the other hand, implies something done together and requires active participation by both parties. It thoughtfully identifies problems and explores ways to deal with them. We believe this distinction is important.

Everyone touched by epilepsy needs education and information. Many people have a difficult time coming to terms with the diagnosis of epilepsy, whether for themselves or for their child. For most, the diagnosis is overwhelming. The enormous amount of information initially given is hard for parents and children to comprehend and absorb. Often, they find it difficult to stand back from the immediate situation and achieve a perspective. A counselor may be able to help them sift through the information the physician has provided, to explain it again, perhaps in different terms, and then to help them begin working on a process of coping.

The counselor wants every person with epilepsy to have ownership and control over their disorder. Counselors can't give them complete control over the medical aspects of their disorder, but they can help them to gain the best control possible over the social ramifications of epilepsy and of their own self-image.

Counseling should be part of the initial educational process, not just directed at working out later problems. Preventive counseling should begin at the time of the diagnosis. If the child and the family don't understand that treatment may require trial-and-error medication adjustment, they may lose trust in their child's doctor when other seizures occur.

Counseling is not for everyone. Some don't need it, and some don't want it. If a person or a family doesn't want it, then it will be of no use to them. All you can do is leave the door open for them to go back later. Another possibility is to try to connect a family with another family or a support group. Talking to other parents and other children may be less threatening than talking to a member of the treatment team.

All families need to be able to communicate, and a counselor gives both the person with epilepsy and the family an opportunity to do just that. They need to talk about the epilepsy but also about all the other things that affect families, like expectations, fears, responsibilities, restrictions, and feelings about themselves and others.

Counseling and education should involve the child, even a child as young as 5 or 6. It is a disservice to leave them out. Involving children early begins the process of ownership of their condition, which, over the long run, will be important in helping them cope.

The counselor doesn't cope for others. The child, the teenager, the adult, and the family will have to cope for themselves. The counselor is the catalyst, suggesting and teaching the tools to help them achieve the benefits of confidence and independence.

Parents often feel isolated, as if life will never be normal again. One approach to this problem is to begin to get the parents involved with activities outside the home. When prompted, parents recognize that they and their child each need some space. They need begin to focus on themselves, on their spouse, on the other children in the family, at least some of the time.

In a support group, which you can often locate through your local epilepsy association, not only do parents give and get support through talking, but often they set up exchanges, in which another parent, knowledgeable about seizures, will care for your child for half a day or one evening and you can do the same for that family. It's called networking. Remember, if you don't take care of yourself, you can't take care of anyone else.

We live in a difficult time, and the divorce rate is high. When a child with a chronic disability is added to the normal family strains and stresses, families often become even more fragile. Communication between partners and with children becomes even more important. Suffering in silence or blaming or laying guilt can be a prelude to disaster. Communication takes hard work and practice. Group support can help establish lines of communication and bring families closer together. Even when children are spending time in two separate households, it's important to remain in close contact to keep information, medication, and medical history consistent.

A couple of principles need to be emphasized. First, people, particularly parents, have to remember that kids with epilepsy are kids first. You can't ascribe all their problems to epilepsy. Kids fight. They sulk. They rebel. They don't do their chores. Epilepsy is not responsible for such behaviors. Epilepsy can influence and increase the magnitude of problems. But how the child handles the epilepsy and how the parents handle both epilepsy and the child will influence that child's future.

CHAPTER 25

Coping with Substantial Disability

Labels should be applied when they are useful as long as the diagnosis does not interfere with proper treatment. If being called "green" gets you or your child an advantage, then your child looks green to us. If your child is labeled "artistic," and this enables them to receive special art classes, then the label will have been useful. If calling them "intellectually disabled" or "on the autism spectrum" enables your child to receive the special help they need in school, then the label may be useful. Correspondingly, if a child is labeled "normal" but has a learning style that requires special help, then the label "normal" may be a disadvantage. However, labeling them "intellectually disabled" may be a disadvantage if what they have is a specific learning disability, and they just need focused help for that problem. If the label "handicapped" places your child in a large class of children with severe disabilities, then the label may not be useful.

It is also important that your expectations for your child be realistic. Putting a child with a disability in a regular class may or may not be to that child's advantage, depending on the child, the class, the nature of the disability, and the alternatives. Mainstreaming (inclusion of children with special needs in regular classes rather than special classes) has many advantages, but it may be a disadvantage for an individual child. The stresses of inappropriate placements may be overwhelming for some children. Neuropsychologists can really help here to give practical advice about what's best for a particular child.

Remember, you can be the best advocate for your child, but be realistic about your child's needs and about what special labels you wish them to have.

Intellectual Disability

In a child with intellectual disability (ID), seizures may further impair function and therefore require aggressive treatment. Even in the child who is profoundly disabled, seizure control may be possible and, if attained, will result in an improved quality of life for the child and their caretakers.

Commonly Asked Questions

Q. *"If my child has epilepsy, what is the chance of intellectual disability?"*
A. The risk of ID in a child with epilepsy depends primarily on the cause of the epilepsy and to a far lesser extent on the type of seizure itself. A previously normal child who begins to have seizures of unknown cause will virtually never become intellectually disabled. If these seizures are caused by a progressive or degenerative disease, however, the risk of ID is high. Children with developmental delay or neurological handicap seldom become more intellectually disabled when seizures are part of the disorder, although it does occur in some syndromes, such as infantile spasms, electrical status epilepticus of sleep, and Lennox-Gastaut syndrome.

Q. *"I don't believe my child is intellectually disabled; I think his problems are due to all those medicines he's taking. How can I tell for sure?"*
A. Overmedicated children often are sleepy during the day or unsteady; children with intellectual disabilities are neither. The only way to rule out medication as a cause is to decrease or eliminate one drug or all drugs in use. Do not do this on your own. With the advice of your child's physician, you may want to consider tapering medication slowly, decreasing a single type of medication at a time. If, on tapering medicine, your child's function obviously improves, then the problems may have been drug related. You and your physician will have to decide whether the risk of decreasing or changing the medication, as well as the chance

of recurring or worsening seizures, is outweighed by the possible benefit of improved intellectual function.

Q. *"How should I treat my child who has both intellectual disability and epilepsy?"*
A. The answer depends on the child's level of disability, particularly for the child with mild or moderate disability. The natural tendency of most parents and grandparents is to overprotect a child with epilepsy. Yet, overprotection, particularly of a mildly intellectually disabled child, leads to infantilization, ultimately a greater handicap to the child than seizures. It is crucial for such a child to be as independent as possible. Children with disability need every opportunity to achieve their optimal potential.

When your child has multiple problems, such as ID and epilepsy, the family has a lot of compensating to do. With epilepsy alone, you can usually maintain your expectations for your child's future—assuming, of course, that they were realistic to begin with—since most epilepsy can be controlled or outgrown. Even when epilepsy occurs in children with ID, your expectations (if well grounded) for your child should rarely be changed.

Helping your child to cope with ID depends greatly on the degree of disability. Severely affected children may not be clearly aware of their disability. Today, many individuals with mild ID and some with moderate intellectual disability function in noncompetitive employment, are able to live in the community with assistance, and engage in various social activities. The process of developing these capabilities begins in childhood, with mainstreaming in schools and socialization through churches, scouting, and athletics. Developing these capabilities begins within the family as well, seeing children's potential, encouraging them to learn to participate, and helping them to achieve their full potential.

Cerebral Palsy
Cerebral palsy (CP) is a group of permanent disorders of the development of movement and posture, causing activity limitations attributed to nonprogressive disturbances that occurred in the developing fetal or

infant brain. It is not caused by a tumor or by degeneration of the nervous system. Cerebral palsy is not progressive—it does not continue to become worse—although it may become more obvious, or its symptoms may vary slightly as the child matures.

Q. *"How can I help my child who has cerebral palsy?"*
A. How you help your child cope with cerebral palsy depends on whether there is also intellectual disability. Many children with cerebral palsy are of normal intelligence, and for these children, the motor dysfunction can be enormously frustrating. To be unable to dress or go to the bathroom alone or to feed oneself can create such a sense of helplessness and dependence that depression is not uncommon among such children. And yet children with cerebral palsy are increasingly able to find areas in which they can become competent and ultimately develop self-esteem. Appropriate use of computers assists learning and communication. Motorized wheelchairs and special adaptations may permit mobility and independence. In addition, therapies and surgeries are being developed to improve muscle tone and the ability to move, and these should be investigated. It is amazing what can be done to help unlock the real person within these disabled bodies.

For the child with cerebral palsy, as for the child with ID, the most important ingredients in successfully adapting are motivation and self-esteem. Motivation can be stimulated by hard work and activities, such as those involved in preparing for the Special Olympics. The joy of successfully participating in sports promotes self-esteem. The Special Olympics are a model of what can be achieved in other areas of life, with patience and persistence. Such children need role models of successful disabled adults. Their ability to become achieving adults begins with small successes in the family and in the school.

Helping your child who has a disability to cope with the accompanying psychological problems is still an art, not a science. There is no how-to manual, although there are many sources of help. Your child and you will need help in articulating your frustrations and concerns, your anger and your hopes.

There has been amazing progress in recent years in enabling both intellectually disabled persons and those with cerebral palsy to participate more fully in the community. The old stereotypes of institutionalization and "handicap" persist, but these children, while *dis*abled, are not *un*able.

Really Difficult-to-Control Seizures

For most children, seizures are not uncontrollable; they are only difficult to control. There is good reason to hope for control. The next medicine may be successful, or a combination of medications may bring control. The ketogenic diet, neurostimulation, or surgery may offer a solution. You may need to get a second opinion, and you may decide to consult with an epilepsy specialist or an epilepsy center. Many times, parents of children with difficult-to-control seizures who persisted in looking for a different therapy turned "uncontrollable" seizures into controlled seizures.

Margo was a bright 10-year-old with intractable seizures. Her hemiparesis was not disabling, but several seizures each week and the effects of all her medications were interfering with her progress. She came to us looking for surgery to remove the epileptic focus. Unfortunately, we found that there were abnormal areas on both sides of the brain, so surgery was not an option. She had had good trials of virtually all the anticonvulsants. After a lot of discussion with her parents and with her, and despite her age, we decided to try the ketogenic diet. Margo said she would do almost anything to get rid of those darn seizures. Margo faithfully stuck to the diet. She had no seizures. After two years on the diet, it was gradually stopped. It's been more than ten years now; Margo is seizure- and medication-free and doing superbly well. She says the diet was really tough but worth it. She has gone on to college, is an amazing author, and is an active volunteer with her local epilepsy association.

Families need to persist in looking for a solution, and physicians also need to be willing to keep trying. Both need to be willing to take risks to achieve benefits. Unfortunately, not every family finds such a happy ending.

Greg is a 15-year-old boy whose seizures began in very early childhood. Although his development was delayed, seizures came under control with medication, and the family came to accept their mildly intellectually disabled son. Genetic testing was done, and no abnormalities were found. At age 5, the seizures recurred, and Greg appeared to become more severely delayed developmentally. The family again went through grieving, anger, and frustration while the physicians tried new medications. Eventually the seizures were again controlled, and the family readjusted to their new circumstances. At age 9, atonic seizures began, and Greg made frequent trips to the emergency room for sutures because of falls. During the brief periods when these seizures were brought under control, Greg could function in the moderately intellectually disabled range, but the frequency of seizures or the side effects of medication continued to be problematic. Repeated genetic testing was done, and still no abnormality was detected. An abnormality on the MRI scan led us to hope that surgery might control his seizures. Surgery was successful, even though his minimal hemiparesis increased. Greg had only rare seizures, in his sleep—at least he wasn't falling—and his language and function improved. Both his family and Greg were delighted. This honeymoon lasted for 6 months, then the seizures recurred. Other therapeutic interventions include a vagus nerve stimulator and perhaps further investigation of surgery for either a corpus callosotomy, further resection, or placement of a responsive neurostimulator. The family went for a second opinion to another epilepsy center, but they didn't have any additional recommendations to make.

In Greg's case, we and the family have a dilemma. We know of no other combination of medicines likely to control his seizures, although there is the continuing promise of new medications being developed. Will further surgery be of benefit? Are the risks of new surgery worth taking? What are the chances of success? The answers are unclear.

There are many lessons in Greg's story. One lesson is that even if parents develop a realistic acceptance of their child's limitations, that acceptance may be challenged when the situation changes. For those families whose children have multiple disabilities, adjustment may be a roller coaster. A second lesson is that often trying a new approach might succeed in controlling intractable seizures. Deciding whether to take the risks of these new approaches when you don't know their benefits in advance can be difficult for both the family and the concerned physician.

There may be a time when you and your child's physician must accept the status quo, but the question will be, when has that time come? Not all our stories have a happy ending.

Coping with Severe Disability and Epilepsy

Parents may come to accept the limitations, even the severe limitations, of their child's cerebral palsy or intellectual disability, realizing that there is no medicine or surgery that can reverse the condition. "But if you could only get rid of the seizures," they may say to us, "life would not be so difficult. I thought you could control seizures with medicine for most children. Why is my child still having seizures?"

Seizures in a child who has other evidence of brain damage or one of the severe genetic abnormalities may be much more difficult to control. Still, your physician should try new medications, the ketogenic diet, or vagus nerve stimulation; and even if your child is intellectually disabled, surgery may not be impossible. You may need to find a physician who is willing to consider new options.

If your child's abnormality is primarily in one portion of the brain, removal of that portion could be of benefit. Most children who are intellectually disabled, however, have damage on both sides of the brain; removal of one portion will not help. Still, even in the child who has bilateral brain damage, vagus nerve stimulation or, rarely, section of the corpus callosum can sometimes help in controlling the atonic or drop seizures that lead to injury.

We treat seizures because they interfere with a child's function. We also know that uncontrolled seizures, especially in sleep, are a risk factor for sudden unexpected death in epilepsy (SUDEP). For the otherwise normal child, occasional seizures that interfere with function require treatment. For the severely disabled child, however, an occasional seizure may be less handicapping than the toxicity of medications. The risks of treatment and its potential benefits must, therefore, be evaluated carefully in light of your child's other disabilities and how closely they are being observed or monitored. When seizures interfere with your child's behavior or function, every reasonable effort should be made to control them.

Parents also often find that it is difficult to obtain childcare for their children with severe disabilities. The CDC has an excellent website that provides information on various services ("Links to Other Websites on Developmental Disabilities," CDC, https://www.cdc.gov/ncbddd/developmentaldisabilities/links.html). In addition, most states have a developmental disabilities administration that can help find local services. Finally, depending on your child's individual diagnosis, many disease- or disability-oriented organizations are also a good resource for help.

Katie was 18 months old and had significant disabilities. She functioned like a 1-year-old. She was not able to walk or talk. Fortunately, her local school system had a superb program for children with disabilities. This program had occupational therapists, physical therapists, and speech therapists. Katie was an ideal candidate—except for her seizures. The school claimed that they had no one who could cope with her frequent generalized tonic-clonic seizures. What would happen if a seizure was prolonged? What were they to do? Katie would require far more time than the other children, and if a seizure occurred, they had no one with the special training needed. Katie's mother had no problem coping with her child's seizures, although she had had no special training. To put it frankly, the school was afraid of accepting the responsibility. Katie was deprived of her right to an optimal program. The school's solution was a home teaching program with visits several times a week. Clearly this was not optimal. Finally, we helped Katie's mother achieve a compromise. She agreed to go to school to handle the seizures while the teachers taught. Over several weeks, the school came to realize that Katie's seizures did not pose a major problem and no longer required that her mother be present. The end of this chapter in Katie's story is that she was found to be a candidate for surgery, her damaged hemisphere was removed, and she no longer has seizures.

A Parent's Special Needs

As parent of a child with severe disability, you have special needs as well. We have talked about success stories, about children who have been cured of their seizures. Magazines are full of such success stories. The epilepsy movement has concentrated on a message of hope in its campaign to eliminate the stigma associated with epilepsy. But for parents of children with significant disabilities or intractable seizures, the message of hope is frustrating. These parents feel left out of the mainstream. They are angry, worried that their children will not get the help they need, and fearful that they themselves will be unable to cope.

Q. *My god! How do I cope with all this?"*
A. You need help! Every parent in a situation like this needs help. Each faces a terrible feeling of loneliness when confronted with the overwhelming dual problems, for example, of intellectual disability and epilepsy. The initial stages of grieving, denial, and anger that any parent with a disabled child experiences are compounded by a feeling of shame, of wanting to tell no one, of feeling that you are the only person in the world who has faced such overwhelming problems. Nor do you want to bother your child's physician with your sense of hopelessness. "He is always so busy." Or maybe the way the physician has explained things to you has simply confused you. "Did she really say . . . ? "

There are several places to turn. First, give your child's doctor another chance. Ask them to explain again. Write down your questions before the appointment; in the stress and intimidation of an office visit, anyone can forget what questions they wanted to ask. A second place to turn is the local affiliate of the Epilepsy Foundation. There are many such affiliates around the country. If you have difficulty finding one, contact the national office of the Epilepsy Foundation in Landover, Maryland. Their toll-free number is 1-800-EFA-1000. For Spanish speakers, the number is 1-866-748-8008. Online, their address is epilepsy.com.

A third and important step is to contact a local support group. Since your child has intellectual disability or cerebral palsy as well as epilepsy, a local organization for intellectually disabled citizens or for individuals with cerebral palsy can be immensely helpful. Many have online support groups that you can participate in virtually.

Q. *"I don't want to be a part of a group. I don't need them, and I don't need to hear about someone else's problems. I have enough of my own."*
A. We often hear this statement from parents. Or else one parent will say, "I'd like to go, but my husband [wife] won't have anything to do with

it." Groups are generally helpful, but some people are just not ready to join a group at a particular time in their lives. Some people are embarrassed to talk about their feelings or problems in public. But you are not the only one who has had to deal with such problems. Hearing how other parents have coped is often far more helpful than hearing similar advice from your child's physician. Parents choose different words, have a different tone to what they say. And they have lived it, not just learned about it. Talking about your problems can help put them in perspective. Recently, there has been an evolution of group meetings online, and this might be helpful to some people who could feel slightly less intimidated.

For the child who has cerebral palsy, and for the parent of that child, United Cerebral Palsy (UCP) provides excellent support services with appropriate guidance and advice. The Arc can provide similar services for the intellectually disabled child and their family. Parents' groups sponsored by these organizations talk about managing intellectually disability or coping with cerebral palsy. They don't talk about seizures, and for parents of children who have intractable seizures, even when ID and cerebral palsy coexist, the focus is often on the seizures. "If only the seizures were controlled, it would be easier to deal with the other problems," such parents often say. It's important for you to decide what is really most important for your child. Maybe it is the seizures. But maybe it isn't. For some children, the problems of intellectual disability are far more important than the seizures. For some children with cerebral palsy, mobility may be the principal problem. For parents of these children, UCP or the local Arc may provide the most important resources. If seizures are the central problem, you may need to educate these organizations about epilepsy and about the special needs of children who have recurring seizures.

The medical community has also failed to serve this population well. This has improved greatly in recent years, since developmental pediatricians are now trained more in child neurology. Developmental pediatricians are trained to help manage the multiple problems of the disabled child and to help families find needed services, but they may have less expertise in epilepsy than in other conditions. Further, neurologists and epileptologists who specialize in treating children's seizures often have inadequate expertise in managing family problems and in finding services. We need to develop better one-stop shopping for this comprehensive care. But until we do, parents of a child with multiple handicaps must continue to advocate and seek services with persistence and determination.

If you feel you do not need a group or feel that you can't cope with counseling just now, reconsider it later. Remember: If you have adjusted so well that you don't need any help, perhaps you are the person who can help someone else.

Coping with Shattered Expectations

Parents of a newborn child have great expectations. These expectations are dashed when a child is diagnosed as having multiple severe handicaps. But such a diagnosis should not mean that all expectations for your child must be abandoned. It means that your expectations must be modified, although your hopes may persist. Parents often tell us that their child's physician had said that their child would never walk. Their child is now walking, and they are angry that the doctor underestimated their child's abilities. Others are angry because their child's physician did not tell them that their child would have troubles in school or be intellectually disabled. When a child is only 1 year old, it may be difficult to predict how well they will talk, walk, or learn. When your child is 3, their doctor may be able to make more precise predictions. By the time your child turns 8, you and your child's physician will have a much better idea about learning problems. The more severely handicapped the child, the earlier accurate predictions can be made.

When you recognize that your child is delayed, make certain that the child's physician explains what is known—and what is uncertain—in terms that you can understand. Don't be afraid to ask questions. When you have recovered from the initial shock, write down or put on a smartphone note any new questions that come to mind and then make another appointment to continue the discussion. Do not hesitate to ask for a referral to another physician for a second opinion. Any physician who refuses or discourages such a second opinion is probably providing a good reason to obtain one. You should remember that a misunderstanding may not be because of what the physician said or didn't say, but rather because of what you heard or didn't hear. No one likes to hear bad news, and we often forget or deny it. In contrast, some people focus on the bad news, ignoring the hopeful signs.

We see so many parents who are trying to obtain the "best" services for their child, but in doing so, they only wear themselves out and exhaust their resources. Occupational therapy to improve feeding on Tuesday and Thursday afternoons, speech therapy Wednesday and Friday, sensory integration therapy Monday and Wednesday mornings. All this for a child who is only 7 months old.

- "If there were only more hours in the day, we could get more therapy and he would start to walk."

- "I know he's only 1 year old, but he's not talking. He needs more speech therapy."

- "The therapist said that she lacks sensory integration and needs therapy."

- "What about the Institute for the Development of Human Potential?"

The learning process is like a bottle with a narrow neck. You can only pour in so much so fast. Despite your desire to do more, you can do only so much, and things can progress only so fast. Development goes at its own pace, and therapy can only help a person around roadblocks. Therapists may help you and your child find a way to solve a problem that was preventing some function: an adapted spoon may make it possible for children to feed themselves, for example. Therapy cannot make development go faster, but specific therapies introduced at the developmentally appropriate stage can be very useful. You wouldn't obtain speech therapy for your normal 10-month-old to help them talk sooner. If your child is developmentally at a 10-month-old level, speech therapy is not going to help them talk until they are ready. Gait training is not useful until the child has achieved the ability to sit and stand. Often it is better when therapists see the child only once a week, or once every two weeks, and teach you how to interact with your child. Then you can provide the therapy several times each day, as you play with your child. Therapists are used most effectively when there is a specific, realistic goal to be achieved.

There may come a time when neither you nor your child's physician can do anything different, or anything more than you are doing. There may come a time to stop your search for the physician who will tell you what you want to hear, for the school that will provide the perfect services and the ideal program for your child. The time may come when you have to accept that you are a good parent, you have been a good advocate for your child, and you have done your best.

No child stays the same forever. All children make progress. In a brain-damaged child, the rate of that progress is a measure of the severity of the neurological damage. For the parents of a child who is profoundly disabled, progress may be measured in terms of smiling, feeding, head control, or reaching—or even just an awareness that you are there. These milestones that parents of more typical children take for granted can be major achievements for children who are profoundly disabled and their families. When your child has severe disabilities, it may be difficult to hold great expectations for the future. Take pleasure in small accomplishments; deal with the bad things, and then set them aside. If you cope in small ways, day by day and week by week, coping in general will become easier. There are many websites with helpful advice and wisdom from other parents that may help you gain perspective. These include the poem "Welcome to Holland" by Emily Perl Kingsley and a lovely haiku by seventeenth-century Japanese poet Mizuta Masahide:

Since my house burned down
I now own a better view
of the rising moon

Perhaps you will be able to see the wonderful child you do have if you can see beyond the old image that you have held in your mind and heart.

Conclusion

You may have read this book for many reasons. Perhaps you were shocked, upset, or disheartened because your child or grandchild has had a seizure or because they have been diagnosed as having epilepsy. Maybe you simply wanted to know more about seizures, their treatment, and what they might do to your child. Whatever the reason, we hope that now you realize that epilepsy is not just a simple medical problem but affects many other aspects of your child's life and your life. We are hopeful that now, more familiar with what epilepsy is and what it is not, you will be able to raise your child in a far more realistic and perhaps optimistic and accepting fashion. It is our hope that your child grows up without disability, or with as few problems as possible, and that you accept them for whatever they may be, help your child fulfill their genuine potential, and not create a situation that limits them unnecessarily.

We hope that you have sensed our own personal involvement with each of our patients, that as you have read the stories of these children, you have sensed how each of the children has affected us, too. We have learned from each of them, and we believe that you can as well. We know that you and your child will find your own ways of coping. Acceptance of seizures and their uncertainties, or of associated learning, motor, or behavioral conditions, does not come easily. And acceptance does not mean resignation. Optimism may at times be hard to find, but it is essential. We strongly believe that our positive approach is realistic. After all, most epilepsy will be controlled, and many children will outgrow it. Even some of the toughest cases can find help, a treatment approach that balances seizures and side effects, and in many cases, a complete end to seizures. It would be a pity if anxiety and overprotection left your child truly disabled or limited in their approach to life. To achieve a full and optimal life, you and your child must both become active, informed, positive participants. We hope that this book has helped and that your child will live a healthy, full, seizure-free life. In the years since the earlier editions of this book were published, we have received hundreds of letters, emails, and phone calls from parents expressing their thanks for our making this information and philosophy available. We wish to express our heartfelt thanks, in return, to all of you who have communicated with us. Your words of appreciation have inspired us to update our book, to add new voices, and to continue our efforts on behalf of children with epilepsy and their families. Our philosophy is optimistic. We hope we have helped you to see the glass as mostly full, to keep your own hopes high, and to set the goals for your child realistically.

We wish you and your child well.

Glossary

absence seizure. A generalized seizure in which consciousness is altered, formerly called *petit mal*, a term no longer used. These seizures are usually brief and occur many times in a day. The EEG pattern is three-per-second spikes and waves. Absence seizures usually respond well to medication and usually are outgrown.

ambulatory monitoring. The use of a wearable, portable EEG device while an individual is awake and at work, school, or play. The ambulatory monitoring device permits prolonged EEG recording during a child's routine activities. Since either the child or another observer must mark events thought to be seizures, and because the amount of EEG information is limited, ambulatory monitoring is typically useful in situations when it is important to clarify the nature of the spell (e.g., faint vs. seizure) and when quantification of spells is important. The procedure is far less expensive than video-EEG monitoring but frequently also less definitive because of the inability for clinical staff (e.g., nurses, EMU technicians) to interact with the patient during an event.

antiseizure medication (ASM). Also called anticonvulsant drug or antiepileptic drug in older literature. A medication used to prevent recurrence of seizures. The particular drug chosen for a child depends on the type of seizures, the age of the child, and the type of side effects that might be expected.

association cortex. The part of the brain in the parietal lobe where vision, hearing, memories, and motor function come together and where there is an integration of information between areas of the brain responsible for sensations, movements, and thoughts.

atonic seizure. A form of generalized seizure in which body tone is suddenly lost and the child slumps to the ground or their head slumps forward. These difficult-to-control seizures often occur in Lennox-Gastaut syndrome. They may resemble the sudden seizure in which the child is thrown to the ground, often injuring the face or teeth. Atonic seizures and myoclonic seizures often occur in the same child, and the terms are often used interchangeably.

atypical absence seizure. A staring spell similar to an absence seizure but often with an atypical EEG. It may last longer than the typical absence seizure and may have other additional features (movement, falling, etc.). Atypical absence seizures may be more difficult to control with medications than typical absence seizures. They are sometimes confused with focal impaired awareness seizures.

aura. The start of a small focal seizure, as recalled by a patient. It may be an abnormal smell, taste, abdominal sensation, or emotion.

automatism. The complex and purposeless automatic movements that accompany a focal impaired awareness seizure. These movements often consist of smacking of the lips, chewing, picking at clothes, or wandering around in a confused fashion.

autonomic nervous system. The part of the brain that controls functions like heart rate, blood pressure, skin temperature, and skin blood flow. Seizures involving the temporal lobe can produce disturbances of autonomic function.

axon. The part of a neuron that resembles an electrical wire and is responsible for the capacity of brain cells to connect and communicate with one another.

breath-holding spell. See *cyanotic breath-holding spell* and *pallid breath-holding spell.*

childhood epilepsy with centrotemporal spikes. The most prevalent epilepsy syndrome of childhood. This was previously called benign childhood epilepsy with centrotemporal spikes (BCECTS) or benign rolandic epilepsy. The seizure often begins with a sensation in the corner of the mouth, followed by local jerking of the muscles; it spreads to one side of the face, or one side of the body, and may become a generalized seizure. It has a typical EEG pattern. These seizures occur more commonly during certain stages of sleep. They are typically outgrown and are usually well controlled with medication.

clonic seizure. The rhythmic jerking of an extremity or the whole body. Seizures that are only clonic are rare. Usually, a seizure starts with tonic stiffening then progresses to clonic movements.

consciousness. Alertness or awareness, the ability to interact normally with the environment. Consciousness is altered in generalized seizures and in focal seizures with impaired awareness but is usually not affected in focal aware seizures.

convulsion. An older term for a seizure. It usually refers to seizures that have a motor component—jerking or stiffening. Other old terms for convulsion include *spell* and *fit*.

convulsive syncope. A seizure that occurs in association with a fainting spell. The child experiences sweatiness, pallor, and dizziness, and faints and loses consciousness. A small percentage of people who faint will then have a brief tonic-clonic seizure. The fainting spell is termed *syncope*; when a tonic-clonic seizure is associated with it, it is called *convulsive syncope*. The convulsion of convulsive syncope is a benign seizure and does not require treatment.

CT (or CAT) scan. Computerized tomography (or computerized axial tomography) uses small doses of X-rays and computer analysis to produce a picture of the brain and enable the physician to see certain abnormalities.

cyanotic breath-holding spell. Breath-holding spells in which the child starts to cry then holds his breath and turns blue before losing consciousness. A seizure occasionally follows a breath-holding spell.

cysticercosis. An infection of the brain caused by a worm that causes cysts within the brain to become calcified and cause seizures. It is more common in low- and middle-income than in higher-income countries.

déjà vu. A sensation that you have seen something or someone before, whether or not you have. This sensation is normal and common, but when it occurs repeatedly, it can be a manifestation of focal seizures starting from the temporal lobe.

dysgenesis. An abnormality of the development of the brain (*dys* = abnormal, *genesis* = creation). There are many different possible abnormalities of cortical development, some of which may cause epilepsy. If the area of dysgenesis is in a place where it may be removed without causing deficit, surgery may cure the seizures.

EEG. The electroencephalogram records the electrical activity of the brain, or "brain waves." The EEG does not provide a diagnosis of epilepsy, but it assists physicians in clarifying the type or origin of seizures.

EEG slowing. Brain activity typically slows during sleep, and this change in frequency can be measured. The amount of slowing can also depend on the age of the child. If the amount of slowing is excessive, or if it is only over one area, it can mean that area of the brain is not functioning normally.

encephalitis. Inflammation of the brain substance itself, due to an autoimmune reaction, or to a bacterial or viral infection.

epilepsies. Seizure patterns whose clinical manifestations and EEGs are sufficiently characteristic for a physician to be able to predict a patient's future course and to recommend specific medications. The term *epilepsies* is also used to indicate that there are diverse forms of repeated seizures (epilepsy), not just one single type.

epilepsy. The term epilepsy is used when a person has experienced two or more unprovoked seizures more than 24 hours apart, or a single seizure with more than a 60 percent chance of recurrence, or the diagnosis of an epilepsy syndrome.

epilepsy syndrome. When features of a child's epilepsy match those of other children with similar seizure types(s), age of onset, EEG findings, responsiveness to certain medicines or other treatments, and other aspects.

epileptogenic. Susceptible to a seizure. Areas of the brain more susceptible to seizures than other areas are considered epileptogenic. The temporal and frontal lobes are usually more epileptogenic than other regions. Certain abnormalities are also considered to be epileptogenic (the areas near scar tissue from an injury, for example).

febrile seizure. A seizure caused by fever. Febrile seizures are common in young children under age 5 because of the lower seizure threshold of the young brain. Only rarely are they associated with later epilepsy. While frightening, they appear to cause little harm. They tend to occur in families. Physicians generally do not prescribe antiseizure medication to prevent these seizures because they are so infrequent (and the treatment is typically not worth it).

focal aware seizures. There is no loss of awareness in this type of seizure. They typically involve motor or sensory symptoms.

focal impaired awareness seizures. During these seizures, the child may stare blankly, then wander, pick at their clothes, do repetitive movements, and appear confused. They last longer than absence seizures.

focal resection. Surgical removal of one area or region of the brain.

focal seizures. Seizures that begin in one part of the brain. Since each area has particular functions, the type of seizure depends on which region is affected. Some are motor, involving the face, hand, or leg; some sensory, involving individual sensations in a part of the body; those involving a temporal lobe produce smells, tastes, fears, or memories, as well as difficulty speaking or understanding someone.

focus. An area of abnormality in the brain responsible for the beginning of a seizure. It is usually determined by EEG (as spikes, sharp waves, or slowing), but a focus could also be suggested by MRI, MEG or PET scan. These local abnormalities may be seen as spikes, or sharp waves, or as slowing on an EEG.

generalized seizure. Seizures that seem to start over diffuse areas of the brain on both sides all at once.

grand mal seizure. The old term for a generalized tonic-clonic seizure. It is no longer used.

half-life. The amount of time it takes for one half of the medication in the body to be metabolized and excreted. This number is used to determine how many times a day a medicine needs to be taken.

hemispherectomy/hemispherotomy. Surgical removal or disconnection (partial removal) of one half of the brain.

hyperventilate. To over-breathe. A physician may instruct your child to take several deep, rapid breaths for 2 to 4 minutes. This overventilation may cause an absence seizure, which can then be observed by your child's doctor. Increased breathing needed during exercise is not the same thing and doesn't cause seizures. Anxiety may cause an individual to hyperventilate. This is also frequently done during outpatient EEG sessions.

hypsarrhythmia. A term used to describe the EEG frequently seen in children who have had infantile spasms. This characteristic EEG pattern is wildly chaotic, of very high voltage, with many spikes and slow waves. The terms *hypsarrhythmia* and *infantile spasms* are often, although incorrectly, used interchangeably. Hypsarrhythmia is the EEG pattern; spasm is the seizure type.

ictus. A Latin term for "stroke" or "blow." A seizure, of whatever type, can be referred to as an ictus as well.

idiopathic. Of unknown cause. Seizures are called idiopathic seizures if no cause can be found. Idiopathic seizures often have a better outcome than those in which a cause is found (genetics or a lesion in the brain). Some also use the word *cryptogenic* to express the same idea—cause hidden or unknown.

infantile spasms (West syndrome). A special form of epilepsy that can occur in the first two years of life from multiple causes. This form of epilepsy is commonly associated with significant intellectual disability and requires prompt diagnosis and treatment with specific medication. The spasms typically disappear by the second to fourth year of life.

intensive monitoring. Monitoring, using modern technology, of the characteristics of an individual's seizures and their correlation with an EEG. Monitoring may include ambulatory monitoring, prolonged EEGs, prolonged video-EEG monitoring, and use of depth electrodes, an electrode grid, or stereoelectroencephalography.

interictal. Describes the period between episodes or seizures. Sometimes, interictal abnormalities can help to diagnose seizure types, even if there is no seizure recorded on the EEG. (See *ictus.*)

juvenile myoclonic epilepsy (JME). A syndrome that begins in late childhood with mild myoclonic jerks on going to sleep or awakening. This jerking may precede or be associated with absence seizures or generalized tonic-clonic seizures. It is often made worse by sleep deprivation and commonly runs in families. JME has a characteristic EEG pattern, and it is generally not outgrown.

Lennox-Gastaut syndrome. A condition that includes two or more types of seizures, one of which is a type in which the child suddenly falls to the ground, often injuring themselves. Absence seizures and generalized tonic-clonic seizures, occurring particularly at night, are common. The EEG shows diffuse spike or polyspike and slow waves. Intellectual disability is common. This is a severe epilepsy syndrome, and one that is difficult to control.

lobes. Parts of the brain. The principal lobes are the frontal lobes, important for motor function, personality, executive function, and memory; the temporal lobes, which are responsible for speech, memory, and emotion; the parietal lobes, which integrate sensory function; and the occipital lobes, which process vision.

megalencephaly. Enlargement of the brain. Abnormalities of brain development may result in brain enlargement. When only one side of the brain is maldeveloped and enlarged (unilateral megalencephaly) and when the child has difficult-to-control seizures, a hemispherectomy may be useful.

meningitis. Inflammation of the coverings of the brain, the meninges. Caused by infectious diseases, meningitis may be accompanied by inflammation of the brain itself (encephalitis), resulting, on occasion, in seizures or brain damage.

migraine. Migraine headaches are characteristically accompanied by paleness, nausea, vomiting, and sleep. They often last more than an hour. On rare occasions they can be confused with or associated with seizures. They tend to run in families.

MRI scan. Magnetic resonance imaging scans, like CT scans, are used to identify structure and abnormalities within the brain. This technique does not use X-rays and gives a clearer picture of brain structure than does the CT scan. It is more expensive and takes longer to do than the CT scan. It also requires that the child remain very still.

myoclonic jerk. Sudden movement of arms or legs, most commonly occurring when a person is falling asleep. Myoclonic jerks during the day may be normal but if frequent could be part of one of the epilepsies.

myoclonic seizure. Abrupt jerks of muscle groups. These jerks may be of a hand, a leg, a shoulder, or sudden flexion of the body forward or backward. While occasional myoclonic jerks may be normal, repeated myoclonic jerks can be a difficult-to-control form of epilepsy; however, not all myoclonus is caused by epilepsy.

neurons. The nerve cells of the brain.

neurotransmitter. The chemicals released by the end (terminal) of an axon into the synapse (the space between neurons). They float across the synapse, or space between cells, and affect the firing of the next cell. Neurotransmitters may have an excitatory or inhibitory effect on the next cell.

pallid breath-holding spell. A sudden loss of consciousness due to slowing of the heart, usually occurring after mild trauma. It may, on occasion, result in a seizure. It is not epilepsy and rarely requires treatment. These spells are the infant form of fainting when blood is drawn. Infants and young children with these spells are at higher risk for fainting in their teenage years.

photic-sensitive seizure. A seizure caused by flashing lights, such as strobe lights or intermittent shining lights, when, for example, driving through trees or along a fence. Photic stimulation is often done during an EEG to see if abnormal discharges or a seizure occurs. In some photic-sensitive individuals, such stimuli may produce seizures.

postictal. A Latin term meaning "after the seizure." (See *ictus.*) Confusion, sleepiness, or weakness after the seizure is termed postictal since it occurs after the event.

prognosis. Outcome or outlook of a medical condition.

psychogenic nonepileptic seizures (PNES). They used to be called pseudoseizures. Events that resemble seizures but are not caused, as a seizure is, by electrical abnormalities in the brain. PNES may be a child's conscious imitation of seizures but more frequently are a subconscious way of coping with various types of stress. PNES often occur in persons who also have true (epileptic) seizures and may be difficult to differentiate from true seizures.

Rasmussen's syndrome. A rare, progressive condition that is characterized by unilateral seizures and progressive one-sided paralysis. Of unknown cause, this condition is best treated with hemispherectomy or hemispheric disconnection.

seizure. A single episode of abnormal brain firing, causing a person to experience altered neurological function. This may involve abnormal awareness, difficulty talking or understanding speech, rhythmic motor movements, abnormal sensations, or changes in vital signs such as heart rate or breathing rate.

shuddering attacks. These are brief episodes of grimacing and shivering movements in infants that increase with excitement. The child typically continues to play or interact normally after an attack.

sleep myoclonus. Sudden jerks of the body, often as someone is going to sleep. These are normal and are not epilepsy.

spell. A term formerly used to describe a seizure. The term is vague and is often used to refer to a seizure or PNES if the nature of that episode is unknown.

spike. An abnormality on an EEG that indicates an electrical discharge of a small number of neighboring brain cells that are not properly controlled for a moment. Repetitive spikes cause electrical seizures, and the spikes may spread to involve enough brain cells to cause a true change in function or behavior, that is, a clinical seizure.

status epilepticus. A single seizure lasting 5 minutes or longer, or back-to-back seizures within a 30-minute period. This definition is intended to bring treatment to a person much more quickly than the previous definition of status epilepticus as a seizure lasting longer than 30 minutes. Status epilepticus can be convulsive or nonconvulsive when a patient is unresponsive but has an ongoing electrical seizure on the EEG.

stereoelectroencephalography. A type of invasive brain monitoring in which thin electrodes are placed in areas of interest in the brain through small holes in the skull.

storage disease. One of the metabolic diseases in which some material, usually a breakdown product of normal tissue, cannot be further metabolized and is stored within nerve cells of the brain. This storage produces malfunction of the cells; it is commonly associated with progressive intellectual and neurological deterioration and with seizures. Each of the various storage diseases has a name.

Sturge-Weber syndrome. A genetic neurocutaneous disorder involving the brain and the skin. Characterized by a birthmark (hemangioma, or port wine stain) involving the forehead and variable parts of the face, often associated with vascular abnormality of the brain, seizures, progressive one-sided weakness, and intellectual disability.

sudden unexpected death in epilepsy (SUDEP). An unexpected, nontraumatic, and non-drowning-related death in a patient with epilepsy.

symptomatic. Indicating a defined cause. Seizures due to fever, meningitis, chemical abnormalities, or head trauma are called symptomatic seizures, or provoked seizures.

synapse. The tiny space between the end of one neuron's axon and the cell body of the next neuron.

syncope. Fainting. The characteristics include a feeling of dizziness associated with pallor and sweatiness, followed by loss of consciousness. When this benign condition is followed by a brief tonic-clonic seizure, it is termed convulsive syncope.

syndrome. A collection of signs or symptoms that together form a condition with a known outcome or that require special treatment.

therapeutic range. The range of medication levels within the blood in which seizures begin to be controlled (lower level) in a majority of patients without toxicity (upper level).

threshold. The susceptibility of a single neuron to fire or of the brain to have a seizure. Many factors may lower the brain threshold and precipitate a seizure. Antiseizure medications raise the threshold and make seizures less likely.

tics. Sudden, episodic, repetitive movements, most commonly involving eye blinking or movements of the face and head, but sometimes other parts of the body. These complex movements are not associated with alterations in consciousness, and they can usually be stopped consciously for a time. They are not associated with EEG abnormalities and are not seizures.

Todd's paralysis. Weakness occurring in one limb or one side of the body after a focal or unilateral seizure. This paralysis, while often thought of as exhaustion of the brain, actually results from inhibition of the seizures and of the normal function of the brain on that side. Todd's paralysis after a seizure is usually resolved in one to two hours but may, on occasion, continue for several days. It always disappears completely.

tonic-clonic seizure. The generalized seizures people often think of when they think of epilepsy, formerly called grand mal seizures. They are characterized by stiffening and then rhythmic jerking movements of the body.

tonic seizure. A seizure that involves stiffening of the arms, legs, and back, as well as a loss of consciousness. The stiffening may last several seconds to a minute. Most tonic seizures go on to a clonic component. Tonic seizures are uncommon except as the first part of the tonic-clonic seizure.

tuberous sclerosis. A genetic disease characterized by abnormal cell development. Because it is caused by abnormal development of cells, lesions can be seen in the brain, eyes, heart, skin, or kidneys.

unilateral seizure. A seizure involving one side of the body, usually the face, arm, or leg. A unilateral seizure involves or spreads through a single half of the brain.

video EEG. The use of video cameras to capture visually the onset and characteristics of seizures or episodes while simultaneously monitoring the EEG to see electrical changes. Video-EEG monitoring permits a physician to identify whether a seizure is associated with an EEG change, that is, whether it is a real (epileptic) seizure or a psychogenic nonepileptic seizure. It will often enable physicians to identify the areas in the brain where the individual's seizures are beginning.

Index

Page numbers with "f" and "t" indicate figures and tables, respectively. Medications are indexed by their generic names (brand names follow in parentheses)

epilepsy: defined, 15, 16t, 124; and febrile seizures, 73–75; iceberg analogy, 15–17, 17f; myths and prejudices, 2–4, 302. *See also specific types*
epilepsy, causes of, 138–56; autoimmune disorders, 143–44; infections, 135–36, 141–42; strokes, 140–41. *See also* genetic changes; genetic predispositions; genetic syndromes
Epilepsy Foundation (EF): camps, workshops, and support groups, 253, 297, 300; consensus statement on seizure-free interval, 260; local affiliates, 253, 294, 297, 300, 322; public education efforts, 3–4; support of alert device research, 265; website resources, 165, 177, 195, 197, 210, 262, 264, 266, 300
epilepsy syndromes, defined, 16t, 124. *See also specific types*
epileptic, as pejorative, 1, 4, 253–54
epileptic aphasia, 133
epileptogenic regions, 28
Equal Employment Opportunity Commission (EEOC), 279
erythromycin, 221–22
ESES (electrical status epilepticus of sleep), 113, 133, 197, 315
eslicarbazepine (Aptiom), 170, 176, 179
estate planning, 270
ethosuximide (Zarontin), 127, 153, 162, 170–71, 173
everolimus, 152
excitation/inhibition balance, 11–12, 12f, 13, 13f
exercise. *See* physical activity
eye movements: artifacts on EEGs, 100f, 104; in nonepileptic events, 63

fainting, 50–51, 52–54, 58, 76
false positives, 264, 265
family. *See* parents and family
fear: sensation of, during seizures, 21, 32, 36, 292; as stage of acceptance, 293–94, 302, 306–7
febrile seizures, 68–75; age as factor, 14, 68, 69; characteristics, 69; common

questions about, 71–75; and Dravet syndrome, 135, 136; evaluation and testing, 68–69, 70–71, 284; risks associated with, overview, 74t; what to do/not do during, 69–70
feelings. *See* emotions
felbamate (Felbatol), 172
fenfluramine (Fintepla), 180
fetal barbiturate syndrome, 276
fetal hydantoin syndrome, 275, 276
fevers, and seizure thresholds, 14, 69, 71. *See also* febrile seizures
financial concerns: estate planning, 270; Medicaid, 269. *See also* insurance
flashing lights, 34–35, 59, 104
focal aware seizures, 22, 32, 35–38
focal impaired awareness seizures: *vs.* absence seizures, 43–45, 110–11; characteristics, 21, 22, 32, 33, 38–39; coping strategies, 292; what to do/not do during, 93–94
focal resection, 206–7, 206f, 319
focal seizures: classification, 22, 23t, 24; defined, 20; and Dravet syndrome, 135; on EEG, 106; localization in the brain, 30–32, 33, 34, 35, 38f, 235; medication for, 170, 171, 173, 174, 175–76, 178, 179, 181; motor or sensory strip localization, 28–29, 37; phases, 21; and Rasmussen's syndrome, 143; recurrence risk, 71, 72, 73, 81; spread of, 25f, 29, 31f, 32, 37–38, 38f, 39, 45; variations, 35–37. *See also* focal aware seizures; focal impaired awareness seizures
focal to bilateral tonic-clonic seizures, 21, 32, 39, 45
folic acid, 276
fosphenytoin, 170
fragile X syndrome, 149
Freeman, John, 186
frontal lobes: as epileptogenic, 28; focal seizures localized in, 33, 38f, 235; structure and function, 9–10, 10f, 26, 26f; surgery on, 204–5
functional MRI (fMRI), 123

Library of Congress Cataloging-in-Publication Data

Names: Vining, Eileen P. G., 1946– author.
Title: Seizures and epilepsy in children : a comprehensive guide / Eileen
P. G. Vining, MD, Sarah C. Doerrer, MS, CPNP, Christa W. Habela, MD,
PhD, Adam L. Hartman, MD, Sarah A. Kelley, MD, Eric H. Kossoff, MD,
Cynthia F. Salorio, PhD, Samata Singhi, MD, MSc, Carl E. Stafstrom, MD, PhD
Description: Fourth edition. | Baltimore : Johns Hopkins University Press,
2022. | Series: A Johns Hopkins Press health book | Revised edition of:
Seizures and epilepsy in childhood : a guide / John M. Freeman, Eileen
P. G. Vining, Diana J. Pillas. 3rd ed. 2002.
Identifiers: LCCN 2022005143 | ISBN 9781421445090 (paperback) | ISBN
9781421445106 (ebook)
Subjects: LCSH: Epilepsy in children—Popular works. | Convulsions in
children—Popular works. | Health education—Popular works.
Classification: LCC RJ496.E6 F7 2022 | DDC 618.92/853—dc23/eng/20220223
LC record available at https://lccn.loc.gov/2022005143

A catalog record for this book is available from the British Library.